POPE PIUS XII LIB., ST. JOSEPH COLLEGE
3 2528 01350 6441

Medical Care and the Health of the Poor

Medical Care and the Health of the Poor

Cornell University Medical College Eighth Conference on Health Policy

EDITED BY

David E. Rogers and Eli Ginzberg

WESTVIEW PRESS

BOULDER • SAN FRANCISCO • OXFORD

Published in 1993 in the United States of America by Westview Press, Inc., 5500 Central Avenue, Boulder, Colorado 80301-2877, and in the United Kingdom by Westview Press, 36 Lonsdale Road, Summertown, Oxford OX2 7EW

Library of Congress Cataloging-in-Publication Data
Cornell University Medical College Conference on Health Policy
(8th : 1992 : New York, N.Y.)
Medical care and the health of the poor / Cornell University Medical College Eighth Conference on Health Policy : edited by David E. Rogers and Eli Ginzberg.
p. cm.
Conference held in New York, N.Y., in 1992.
Includes bibliographical references and index.
ISBN 0-8133-1720-7
1. Poor—Medical care—United States—Congresses. 2. Poor—Health and hygiene—United States—Congresses. I. Rogers, David E. (David Elliot), 1926– . II. Ginzberg, Eli, 1911– . III. Title.
[DNLM: 1. Health Policy—congresses. 2. Health Services—congresses. 3. Medical Indigency—congresses. 4. Poverty—congresses. W 250 C814m 1992]
RA418.5.P6C68 1992
362.1'0425—dc20
DNLM/DLC
for Library of Congress

92-49555
CIP

Printed and bound in the United States of America

The paper used in this publication meets the requirements of the American National Standard for Permanence of Paper for Printed Library Materials Z39.48-1984.

10 9 8 7 6 5 4 3 2 1

Contents

Tables and Figures

Tables

Figures

Introduction

David E. Rogers

Over the past eight years, a series of conferences held at Cornell University Medical College have focused attention on certain problems causing serious pain on the U.S. health care scene. The format of these conferences has been straightforward. A small group of distinguished individuals who have spent their professional lives working on the topic under examination have written provocative papers articulating the issues, their thoughts on what caused the problem, its magnitude, and potential ways to mute or solve it. Those papers have then been circulated to a small but diverse group of equally knowledgeable and committed folk from a panoply of disciplines. Both speaker and participants have then come together at Cornell for a vigorous two-day give-and-take. This has resulted in a short book on the subject that generally contains recommendations for action to address the problem more forcibly.

The conferences, and the publications resulting from them, have been well received and seem to be commanding increasing national attention. The topics reviewed over this period have opened a window on where we are doing poorly as a nation. They have included looks at physician supply, clinical decisionmaking and social values, problems relating to the AIDS epidemic, and most recently the burgeoning hazards that beset high-risk children and adolescents and interfere with their chances of becoming healthy adults.

This year we decided to focus on a deceptively simple issue often felt to be the root cause of the depressing U.S. showing in many indices of health. We titled this conference "Medical Care and the Health of the Poor." I state the title because it was chosen with some care. Although it has long been known that there is a strong and compelling correlation between being poor and being sick, beyond this obvious point causality relationships quickly get murky. To address these relationships, we asked several thoughtful observers of the issues surrounding this correlation to bring us some data. Just how tight is this correlation? Which comes first—poverty or ill health? Which most improves health—income enhancement or more medical care? How does poverty affect access to medical services? More to the point, if a person gets to those services, is health improved or infirmity avoided? How does schooling, housing, occupation, nutrition, or race fit into the picture?

All of our participants have spent considerable amounts of their adult lives working on different facets of this problem. As a matter of fact, I calculated that more than 700 years of collective professional experience regarding these linkages were in the heads of those who participated in the conference.

The dialogue was full of depth and intensity. I hope you, the reader, enjoy the following chapters, Dr. Ginzberg's overview, and my summation of where we left this subject.

1

Overview

Eli Ginzberg

The chapters that follow reproduce the seven invited papers that were prepared for the Cornell University Medical College Eighth Conference on Health Policy on the theme medical care and the health of the poor. Chapter 4 reproduces the speech delivered by the newly appointed commissioner of health in New York City, Dr. Margaret Hamburg, and the book concludes with a summation on the conference by the co-convener, Dr. David Rogers, who emphasizes the policy directions that emerged from the two-day discussion. Despite some differences in emphasis and interpretation, the conferees were in broad agreement as to the directions for policy initiatives.

In this overview chapter I have set myself the task of informing the reader about the principal issues on which the conferees centered their attention, taking care to note both the broad areas of agreement and the issues about which differences were not fully resolved. This overview and the subsequent chapters follow the order in which the several presenters delivered their papers.

Victor Fuchs begins by raising incisive questions about the relationship between poverty and health. He points out the conceptual difficulties one encounters in defining the term *poverty*; what measures of health should be employed—morbidity, mortality, or disability; how such measures differ among age groups in the same country and among countries; and whether the relationship between poverty and health is mediated by such factors as individual differences regarding time preferences and self-efficacy.

Fuchs goes on to raise additional policy questions such as the correlation between specific aspects of poverty and poor health. Do the poor suffer more morbidity and higher mortality because they are unable to obtain ready access to the health care system and quality care? Or is their inferior health status more a reflection of inadequacies in nutrition, housing, and neighborhood conditions? Fuchs also emphasizes the tensions that exist in a democracy such as ours among the drive to greater equity, the resistance of the public to higher taxes, and the societal necessity to pay attention to efficacy in the use of scarce resources.

Paul Starr looks at the politics of health care inequalities. The issue at hand could be reformulated as, "How much inequality in health care can a democratic society tolerate, and how much inequality in access to health care should responsible citizens in a democracy accept?" Starr remarks that most democratic societies have not necessarily committed themselves to broad-based "universalism"; rather, they have been willing to tolerate a considerable degree of inequality in the provision of medical care to different classes. He believes that a reasonable degree of inequality of access can be consistent with the democratic ethos so long as the poor are part of the same broad system of health care available to the rest of the society, even if the wealthy have the option of using their own money to obtain extra care. Starr concludes that if the poor are part of the mainstream system of care, they will enjoy the basic protection against illness that should be available to all citizens in a democracy.

Sir Douglas Black is the author of a well-known 1980 report that examined the relationships between occupational class and health status in Great Britain during the three decades of experience under the National Health Service. That report revealed that while there were notable improvements in the overall long-term trends in mortality and morbidity, the relative standing among the country's five occupational classes had not narrowed, much less disappeared, over the three decades.

In reflecting on this surprising outcome, Black focuses special attention on individuals and families that live in particularly disadvantaged environments. He sees the "social deprivation" that they suffer as the key cause of their inferior health status and dismisses the notion that their poor health is the primary cause of that deprivation.

In seeking leverages for constructive change, Black singles out children as the primary group warranting special attention and assistance since improving their health will have long-term payoffs. He recommends greater safety for children at home and at play to reduce serious accidents and premature death; better nutrition via school meals; and regular assessment and recording of their hearing, vision, height, and weight at school; and health education that discourages cigarette smoking.

Dr. Nicole Lurie looks closely at the experiences of the poor in securing effective treatment for hypertension and diabetes. She notes that because of less education, membership in a stigmatized group, and inadequate insurance coverage, the poor are likely to encounter major barriers to effective diagnosis and treatment.

Focusing primarily on financial barriers, Lurie emphasizes that in the case of chronic conditions in which patients must make use of ongoing medications, many of which have risen substantially in price, if also in efficacy, inadequate money or insurance coverage is a major barrier to optimal care. Although improved insurance coverage would not remove all barriers to optimal care since considerations of race and patient-physician circumstances might still impede the poor obtaining optimal treatment, such an improvement would help increase the quality and effectiveness of the care the poor do receive.

Doctors Mary Charlson, John Allegrante, and Laura Robbins focus on arthritis and its treatment. In doing so, they point out that the poor and the less educated are much more likely to develop arthritis and to develop more severe manifestations of the disease, are less likely to seek treatment, and are less likely if treated to undergo major surgical interventions that can moderate and often cure the condition. What is more, the authors demonstrate that the much higher prevalence and seriousness of the disease among the poor reflect in the first instance the dysfunctional work, much of it involving bending and heavy lifting, that so many of them have earlier performed.

Even if it is difficult in the short and middle term to eliminate the jobs that contribute to disability resulting from arthritis, modern medicine can do much to moderate and remove the dysfunctional consequences of the illness—but only if the poor have broadened access to the health care system. Such broadened access would be cost-effective for society by reducing the long-term costs of care for large numbers of seriously afflicted arthritic patients.

Dr. C. Arden Miller sounds an upbeat note in regard to children's health by stressing that several interventions have proved effective, including income supplementation, newborn screening, family planning, and Head Start. Miller focuses on the latter two interventions. He emphasizes that unwanted or mistimed childbearing is a harbinger of poor pregnancy outcomes and that Americans are conspicuously poor users of contraceptives.

He also remarks that the serious lack of health assessment, surveillance, and treatment for children in the early developmental years who need medical attention and treatment could be addressed by Head Start. It is an ideal instrument for providing such health surveillance of children and for securing parental involvement in their care. To date, however, the program serves only about 20 percent of all poor children. Taxpayers have been unwilling to fund the program at the level that is required. This is an egregious neglect that if overcome could make a significant contribution to improving the health and future opportunities of poor children.

Diane Rowland reviews the aims and successes of both Medicare and Medicaid and emphasizes that each has contributed substantially to broadening the access of the elderly and the poor to health care services. Medicare has come close to being a universal system since almost all of the elderly are covered. Medicaid, however, has never covered more than about two-thirds of the poor and today possibly not much more than half. But even Medicare has its shortcomings: The financially vulnerable elderly have to make substantial co-payments to obtain care, especially if they lack Medigap coverage or are not eligible for Medicaid. Rowland concludes from her in-depth review that improving health care for the poor must include universal financing with adequate benefits.

In my summary I note that although substantial agreement emerged during the conference in favor of a more inclusive system of health care financing and delivery with minimal or no exclusion of any group based on income, location, or other social characteristic, serious barriers still exist to the achievement of this objective in the immediate or near future. In 1965 when the legislation instituting Medicare and Medicaid was passed, total U.S. health care expenditures amounted to $41 billion. They are estimated for calendar 1992 to be around $820 billion and are on their way to $1 trillion by 1994–1995. Projections to the year 2000 point to the necessity of finding a second trillion dollars, which is highly improbable for a $5.5 trillion economy that is growing at 2 to 2.5 percent per annum.

Thus, I voice a caution: Significant improvements in medical care for the poor will require that the more affluent beneficiaries of Medicare accept fewer benefits and/or higher taxes; that those who enjoy both good wages and comprehensive health care benefits forego some or most of the federal tax subsidy that helps finance these benefits; that many acute care hospitals with an average occupancy of slightly more than 60 percent merge, change their mission, or close; that many of the more than 9 million people currently employed in the health care industry find employment in other sectors of the economy; that physicians and other health professionals recognize and accept that their relative earnings will decline; that the well insured accept considerable restrictions on their choice of providers; that government substantially restrict the scope of private health insurance companies; and that the principal payers—government and employers—put in place a system of global budgeting and basic reforms aimed at simplifying the complex and costly administrative superstructure. In the absence of these and still other major reforms, the federal government, whose accumulated deficit has grown from $1 to $4 trillion since the beginning of the 1980s, will be hard-pressed to maintain its present and prospective outlays for Medicare and Medicaid, much less put in place improved coverage for the poor.

The best hope for a significant improvement in the health of the poor rests on a strong and continuing expansion of the U.S. economy accompanied by an expanded program of social reform. The poor need more jobs, more income, more subsidized housing, and better public education as much or more than they need better access to health care. Thirty years separated the Great Society from the New Deal. By the mid-1990s, the country should be ready for a new advance.

2

Poverty and Health: Asking the Right Questions

Victor R. Fuchs

Gertrude Stein, noted author and confidante of the leading writers, artists, and intellectuals of her time, lay dying. Her closest friend and lifetime companion, Alice B. Toklas, leaned forward and said, "Gertrude, what's the answer?" Gertrude looked up and with her last breath said, "Alice, what's the question?"

Regarding the issue of medical care and the health of the poor, we must indeed ask "what is the question?" Or, more appropriately, "what are the questions?" Unfortunately, too often the only questions addressed by writers on health policy are those for which they have predetermined answers. I propose to inject a different perspective by raising several theoretical questions about poverty and health so as to elicit answers that might improve public policy.

Who Are the Poor?

A logical place to begin is by asking what we mean by poverty—that is, who are the poor? This question has a long history within economics and even from the perspective of that single discipline gives rise to considerable controversy over definition and measurement. The question becomes even more important, however, when poverty is discussed in relation to health. As an economic concept, there is general agreement that poverty refers to some measure of income (or wealth) that indicates "inadequate" command over material resources. In the health care field, however, the

---

Comments from Alan Garber, M.D., John Hornberger, M.D., and Douglas Owens, M.D., are gratefully acknowledged.

concept often gets transformed into an amorphous set of "socioeconomic conditions" or an ill-defined "culture of poverty."

Let us try to avoid such confusion. This is not to deny that people can be "poor" in ways other than economic. They can be "spiritually impoverished," "morally bankrupt," "unhealthy," and so on. But to the extent possible, let us strive for clarity. If we mean low income, let us say low income. If we mean education, let us say education. And if we mean alcoholism, cigarette smoking, crime, drug abuse, fragmented families, hazardous occupations, sexual promiscuity, slum housing, social alienation, or unhealthy diets, let us say so explicitly. If we constantly redefine poverty to include anything and everything that contributes to poor health, we will make little progress either in theory or practice.

Even when poverty is defined in terms of income, there are numerous questions still to be answered, such as adjustment for size and composition of household, but we can leave them to the specialists.[1] There is one conceptual issue, however, that is so important as to require explicit discussion. Should poverty be defined according to some fixed standard (absolute income) or according to position in the income distribution (relative income)? In my judgment, we need to combine both approaches. If we cling only to a fixed standard, economic growth gradually raises almost everyone out of poverty so defined, but the problems we usually associate with poverty persist. So-called subsistence budgets are adjusted to new social norms. Alternatively, to define poverty in terms of the bottom 10 or 20 percent of the income distribution does not help us get to the heart of the problem either. In a society with little inequality of income, being at the lower end need not have the same negative implications as when the distribution is very unequal.

People usually think of themselves as poor (and are regarded as poor) when their command over material resources is much less than others. Poverty as an economic concept is largely a matter of economic distance. Thus, in 1965, I proposed a poverty threshold of one-half of median income.[2] The choice of one-half was somewhat arbitrary, but the basic idea would not change if a level of four-tenths or six-tenths was chosen instead.

There is considerable resistance to such a definition because a reduction in poverty so defined requires a change in the distribution of income—always a difficult task for political economy. But I believe it is the only realistic way to think about poverty. In this respect, as in so many others, Adam Smith had a clear view of the matter more than 200 years ago when he wrote, "By necessaries I understand not only the commodities which are indispensably necessary for the support of life but whatever the custom of the country renders it indecent for creditable people even of the lowest order to be without."[3]

What Is the Relation Between Poverty and Health?

Once we have identified the poor, the next question concerns their health relative to the rest of the population. We know in general the answer to this question—on average those with low income have worse health. There are, however, several aspects of the question that deserve further exploration. How does the relation vary with different measures of health, such as morbidity, disability, or mortality? Is the relation different for different diseases? Is it different at different stages of the life cycle? Is the relation stronger in some countries than in others? If any of these questions are answered in the affirmative (and they surely will be), the next step is to determine the reasons for the variation. Such inquiries can provide valuable inputs into the next stage of analysis when we seek to make inferences about causality.

Is Low Income the Cause of Poor Health?

Many writers simply assert, without rigorous testing, that poverty is the cause of poor health. In England, social class is often used as a proxy for poverty, but this is problematic, as illustrated in Table 2.1. There is a large differential in mortality between the lowest and the highest class and a large differential in income as well, but more detailed inspection reveals a complex pattern. Class II has only 5 percent greater mortality than class I, even though income is 23 percent lower. In contrast, the differential in mortality between classes IV and V is 21 percent, but the income difference is only 2 percent. It may be tempting to explain these data by asserting that the relationship between income and mortality is nonlinear. Thus, at low levels of income (classes IV and V) even a small increase in income has a strong effect on mortality, whereas at high levels (classes I and II) the effect is very weak. This explanation will not wash, however, once we note that the mortality differentials between classes I and V were no smaller in 1971 than in 1951. During those two decades, real earnings rose by more than 50 percent for all classes; thus, if nonlinearity is the explanation for the pattern shown in Table 2.1, there should have been an appreciable narrowing in the class mortality differentials between 1951 and 1971. No such decrease occurred. Furthermore, there was no decrease between 1971 and 1981 despite additional increases in real income.

England is not alone in experiencing persistence of class (occupation) differentials in mortality in the face of rising real income and universal coverage for medical care. In Scandinavia, the age-standardized mortality ratio for male hotel, restaurant, and food service workers is double that of teachers and technical workers.[4] A Swedish study of age-standardized death rates among employed men aged forty-five to sixty-four found sub-

TABLE 2.1
Indexes of Mortality and Income in England and Wales by Social Class, 1971 (class I = 100)

Social Class		*Age-Adjusted Mortality, Men 15–64*	*Gross Weekly Income*
I.	Professional	100	100
II.	Managerial	105	77
III.	Skilled	136	58
IV.	Semiskilled	148	51
V.	Unskilled	179	50

Source: Adapted from R. G. Wilkinson, "Socioeconomic Differences in Mortality: Interpreting the Data on Their Size and Trends," in R. G. Wilkinson, ed., *Class and Health: Research and Longitudinal Data* (London: Tavistock, 1986), pp. 2, 11.

stantial differences across occupations in 1966–1970 and slightly greater differentials in 1976–1980.[5] In Sweden, there is growing recognition that these differentials cannot be explained by differential access to health care. Johan Callthorp writes, "There is no systematic evidence that the health care system is inequitable in the sense that those in greater need get less care or that there are barriers towards the lower socioeconomic groups."[6]

What Explains the Correlation Between Poverty and Health?

That variables A and B are correlated does not, of course, prove that A is the cause of B. Two other possibilities must be considered. First, the causality may run in the opposite direction: B may be the cause of A. The possibility that health affects social class has been explored extensively by British writers.[7] Almost all agree that there is some "selective mobility," but no consensus has emerged regarding its importance. R. G. Wilkinson concludes that "its contribution to observed class differences in health is probably always small."[8] But Roy Carr-Hill writes, "There is an effect which should not be ignored: the size of the effect could be substantial, but it cannot be estimated properly without a lifelong longitudinal study."[9]

Second, one or more "third variables" may be the cause both of low income and poor health. These variables could include genetic endowment as well as numerous socioeconomic factors. Among the latter, most U.S. studies have focused on schooling. There is a vast literature that explores the relation between health and education.[10] To be sure, income and education are correlated, but the correlation is not so high as to preclude sorting out their separate relationships with health. In the United States, the coefficient of correlation between education and income within age-sex-race groups never reaches as much as .50 and is typically around .40.

When health is regressed on both income and schooling, the latter variable always dominates the former. Indeed, in some studies income is negatively related to health once years of schooling are controlled for.[11]

Why Is the Correlation Between Schooling and Health So Strong?

One possible answer, of course, is that schooling is the cause of good health. That is, at any given level of income, those with more education know how to use medical care more effectively, choose better diets and other health behaviors, and so on. This line of reasoning has been developed most fully by Michael Grossman.[12] But again, as a matter of logic, we must consider two other possibilities. Good health may lead to more schooling, or there may be third variables that affect both schooling and health. Among the third variables, my favorite candidates are time preference and self-efficacy.[13]

Time preference is an economic concept that refers to the rate at which people discount the future relative to the present. Individuals with high rates of time preference will tend to invest less in the future: On average they will have less education, lower income, and worse health. A perfect capital market would enable those with low rates of time discount to provide funds to those with high rates until their rates were equal at the margin, but the real world bears little resemblance to this theoretical model. For one thing, low-income individuals who want to borrow a great deal cannot provide effective collateral. Also, many choices about health do not involve money; thus, there is no effective market in which individuals with different rates of time preference can make trades.

Self-efficacy is a psychological term that describes people's beliefs in their capability to exercise control over their own behavior and their environment. Differences among individuals in self-efficacy are probably correlated across several domains, such as health and education, thus helping explain the close relationship between these variables.

How Does Low Income Affect Health?

Let us return to the line of inquiry that has poverty as a cause of poor health. Within that framework the central question concerns the mechanism through which low income translates into bad health. To what extent does the health of the poor suffer because they have inadequate access to medical care? To what extent is their poor health the result of deficiencies in other health-producing goods and services such as good food, good housing, and a safe environment? If poor health is attributable to inadequate medical care, are the barriers faced by the poor simply a matter of purchasing power, or are there other impediments?

What Are the Most Important Health Problems Facing the Poor?

In addressing this question, I want to distinguish between relative risk and absolute risk, a distinction that is often obscured in the media and even in policy discussions. For example, infant mortality may be twice as high among the poor as the nonpoor (a relative risk of 2 to 1), whereas the differential in mortality from heart disease may be only 50 percent (a relative risk of 1.5 to 1). The absolute level of risk of infant mortality, however, may be very low relative to heart disease mortality; thus, the poor might benefit more from efforts devoted to heart disease rather than to infant mortality.

To illustrate this point, let us consider the tremendous attention given by the media (and many health policy experts) to black-white differences in infant mortality and the relative neglect of other black-white health differentials. It is true that the black infant death rate is double the white rate, while the difference in overall life expectancy is only 9 percent (75.9 years versus 69.7 years in the United States in 1989). But if the black infant mortality rate was reduced to the white level (and all other age-specific rates remained unchanged), black life expectancy would rise only by six-tenths of a year. More than 90 percent of the black-white difference in life expectancy would remain. Is there not a danger that undue emphasis on attention-grabbing headlines results in a misallocation of health care resources from the perspective of those whose health problems are being addressed?

Which Health Problems of the Poor Are Most Amenable to Solution?

To make rational allocations of resources to alleviate the health problems of the poor, it is necessary but not sufficient to know the relative importance of the problems. It is also necessary to know how readily the problems can be solved or alleviated. Unfortunately, the bulk of health policy research dwells on documenting the problems of the poor, while it neglects the more difficult task of assessing the efficacy of alternative interventions. Policymakers and the public need to know both the costs and benefits of such alternatives. For example, treatment for infectious diseases may be very efficacious, whereas treatment for cancer may not be. Some prevention programs, such as immunizations, may provide a great deal of benefit for little cost, but others, such as mass screening of cholesterol levels, may use a vast amount of resources for limited benefits.

Are There Reasons for Providing Medical Care to the Poor Other Than Improving Health Outcomes?

Suppose the contribution of medical care to health at the margin is quite small. Is that sufficient reason to ignore the provision of care to the poor? Not necessarily. In his critique of the Oregon plan for rationing medical care to the poor, Bruce Vladeck writes, "We expect the health system to take care of sick people whether or not they are going to get better."[14]

Medical care may be valued by the poor (as it is by the nonpoor) for the caring and validation services that it provides. If this is the case, serious questions arise concerning the *kind* of care provided to the poor. In particular, is "high-tech" care overemphasized at the expense of simpler, more valuable services? That medical care has value apart from improving health outcomes provides no grounds for rejecting a cost-benefit approach to resource allocation. But it does highlight the need to incorporate the value of all services in such analyses.

What Policy Instruments Are Available to Help the Poor?

A sociologist tried to explain poverty to a colleague in economics. "You know, the poor are different from you and me." "Yes," replied the economist, "They have less money." This apocryphal exchange highlights a continuing controversy over the best way to help the poor with respect to health or anything else. If more resources are to be allocated to the poor, is it better to provide cash and allow the poor to decide how to spend it, or should the transfers be tied to particular goods and services? The arguments for tied transfers usually derive from a paternalistic assumption that the poor, left to their own devices, will not spend the money "wisely"—that is, they will buy cake when those making the transfers think they should buy bread. A more sophisticated version of this argument invokes "externalities." It may be the case that forcing the poor to spend their additional resources on immunizations rather than on alcohol helps the nonpoor because the former creates positive externalities, whereas the latter creates negative ones.[15] But the same is true of expenditures by the nonpoor.

Paternalism aside, there is the practical question of whether tied transfers can alter consumption patterns. If a family that previously spent $250 per month on food receives $100 worth of food stamps, there is no reason to expect spending on food to rise to $350. Indeed, food expenditures are not likely to increase by any more than if the family received $100 in cash. The relative price of food at the margin is no different after the transfer than before. The only way to assure a disproportionate increase in food consumption would be to provide food stamps greater in amount than what the family would voluntarily spend on food, given its income plus the cash value of the food stamps.

In devising programs for the poor, physicians usually advocate more medical care; educators, more schooling; the construction industry, more housing; and so on. But what area(s) would the poor give highest priority? This question is beyond the scope of this chapter, but it cries out for attention from policy analysts in some setting.

In choosing between in-kind and cash programs, policymakers should also consider the pecuniary effects of alternative transfers to the poor.[16] One result of Medicare and Medicaid, for example, was higher incomes for physicians—surely not a goal of the Great Society. These programs also led to an increase in the price of medical care for the general public, including many low-income persons who did not qualify for Medicaid. If instead of Medicare and Medicaid, the government had transferred to the elderly and the poor an equivalent amount of cash, some of it would have been used for medical care, but much of it would have been used for other goods and services, including food, clothing, consumer durables, and the like. The income and price effects would probably have been very different from those of Medicare and Medicaid and possibly more egalitarian.

Why Are Americans Less Willing Than Others to Subsidize Medical Care for the Poor?

The health policy literature abounds with articles that describe and decry the difficulty faced by poor Americans in obtaining health care. But these articles are typically silent as to why the United States is the only major industrialized country that does not have national health insurance. In 1976, I proposed several answers to this question: distrust of government, the heterogeneity of the population, the weakness of noblesse oblige, and a robust voluntary sector.[17] In a recent article I reappraise these explanations in the light of subsequent political, social, and economic developments.[18] I have a healthy respect for my opinion, but it would be useful to hear other views on this question.

What Is the Most Efficient Way to Provide Medical Care for the Poor?

The debate on this issue is clear-cut. On the one hand are those who want to provide the poor with health insurance and leave it to them to obtain the care they need. On the other hand are those who advocate special programs directly aimed at providing care for the poor. Inasmuch as both approaches have been tried in the United States and abroad, it should be possible to make some judgments about their relative costs and benefits.

Is it acceptable to provide highly cost-effective care for the poor although the care is different from that available to the nonpoor? A good example is prenatal care and delivery of babies. The Maternity Center Association can provide high-quality midwifery service in its childbearing center for less than half of what Medicaid pays for in-hospital normal childbirth.[19] At present, some poor women get the high-cost care, and some get little or no care.

The question of efficient provision of care to the poor is complicated by the fact that there may be gross inefficiencies in care provided to the nonpoor—overtesting, inappropriate surgery, and so on. Should programs for the poor aim at reproducing these misallocations of resources?

What Is "Two-Tier" Medical Care?

Discussions of medical care for the poor frequently invoke the phrase *two-tier medicine*. For strict egalitarians this is a deplorable concept. But others have argued that an explicit two-tier system would serve the U.S. poor better than does the present jumble of services that range from no care (e.g., prenatal) to the most sophisticated (e.g., neonatal intensive). In thinking about this issue, we can note that two-tier systems can vary greatly, as shown in Figure 2.1. In both systems, the people in the first tier receive more and better service than those in the second. But in version A most of the population is in the first tier, and only the poor are in tier two. In version B the proportions are reversed; most of the population is in the second tier, and only the affluent and/or well connected are in tier one.

Version A provides a "safety net"; version B provides an "escape valve." Most Americans tend to associate two-tier medicine with version A; most other countries have opted for version B. Several interesting questions may be posed about these alternative approaches. Do the two versions have different consequences for cost, access, and quality?

For example, consider cost. Suppose per capita expenditures in tier one are identical in the two systems and the same is true for tier two except that in each country they are 50 percent less than tier one. Suppose that in system A 80 percent of the population are in tier one and 20 percent in tier two, and that the proportions are reversed in system B. In that case, the average expenditure per person in system A will be 50 percent greater than in system B.

What political, social, and economic factors lead a country to adopt one version or the other? It seems that individuals who are certain they would

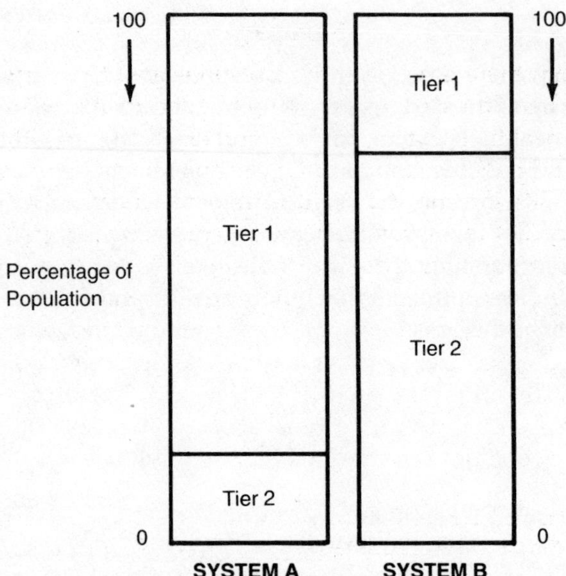

FIGURE 2.1 Two Versions of Two-Tier Medical Care

be in tier two under either system would prefer B. Similarly, individuals who are certain they would be tier one under either system may also prefer B. Supporters of A are likely to be individuals who think they would be in tier one under A but in tier two under B. Many Americans probably fit that category.

What Is Basic Medical Care?

A frequent conclusion of health policy discussions in the United States is that everyone should have access to "basic" medical care. Many observers believe that the nonpoor would be more willing to subsidize a "basic" package than they would complete equality of care. Problems arise, however, in trying to define the contents of that package. Moreover, no matter how they are defined at any point in time, no one should imagine that the contents can remain fixed over time. In a world of changing technology and rising real income, a fixed approach to basic care will prove no more satisfactory than will a fixed poverty standard based on some notion of subsistence. The basic care package will constantly have to change to include "whatever the custom of the country renders it indecent for creditable people, even of the lowest order, to be without."

Summary

In summary, there are numerous questions about poverty and health that need to be addressed. Many of them concern the relation between poverty and health: its extent, pattern, and explanations. Other questions revolve around possible confounding variables such as education, which is correlated with income and health. Still other questions focus on medical care: its efficacy in improving health, its value to the poor, the best way to provide it. In pursuing these questions, we need to find a middle road between a mindless optimism that ignores reality and a constricting pessimism that denies the possibility of creating a more efficient and more just society.

Notes

1. See J. L. Palmer, T. Smeeding, and C. Jenks, "The Uses and Limits of Income Comparisons," in J. L. Palmer, T. Smeeding, and B. Boyle Torrey, eds., *The Vulnerable* (Washington, D.C.: Urban Institute Press, 1988), pp. 9–27.

2. V. R. Fuchs, "Toward a Theory of Poverty," in Task Force on Economic Growth and Opportunity, *The Concept of Poverty* (Washington, D.C.: Chamber of Commerce of the United States, 1965), pp. 71–91.

3. A. Smith, *The Wealth of Nations* (New York: Random House, Modern Library edition, 1937), p. 821.

4. O. Andersen, "Occupational Impacts on Mortality Declines in the Nordic Countries," in W. Lutz, ed., *Future Demographic Trends in Europe and North America* (New York: Academic Press, Harcourt Brace Jovanovich, 1991), p. 46.

5. J. Callthorp, "The 'Swedish Model' under Pressure," *International Journal of Quality Assurance in Health Care* (forthcoming).

6. Callthorp, "The 'Swedish Model'," p. 13.

7. See, for example, A. J. Fox, *Social Class and Occupational Mobility Shortly Before Men Become Fathers*, OPCS Series LS No. 2 (London: HMSO, 1984); J. Stern, "Social Mobility and the Interpretation of Social Class Mortality Differentials," *Journal of Social Policy* 12(1983):27–49; and M. E. J. Wadsworth, "Serious Illness in Childhood and Its Association with Later Life Achievement," in R. G. Wilkinson, ed., *Class and Health: Research and Longitudinal Data* (London: Tavistock, 1986).

8. R. G. Wilkinson, "Socioeconomic Differences in Mortality: Interpreting the Data on Their Size and Trends," in Wilkinson, ed. *Class and Health*, p. 10.

9. R. Carr-Hill, "The Inequalities in Health Debate: A Critical Review of the Issues," *Journal of Social Policy* 16(1987):527.

10. See, for example, M. C. Berger and J. P. Leigh, "Schooling, Self-Selection, and Health," *Journal of Human Resources* 24(1989):435–455; P. Farrell and V. R. Fuchs, "Schooling and Health: The Cigarette Connection," *Journal of Health Economics* 1(1982):217–230; M. Grossman, "The Correlation Between Health and Schooling," in N. E. Terleckyj, ed., *Household Production and Consumption* (New York: Columbia

University Press for NBER, 1976); and D. S. Kenkel, "Health Behavior, Health Knowledge, and Schooling," *Journal of Political Economy* 99(1991):287–304.

11. R. Auster, I. Leveson, and D. Sarachek, "The Production of Health: An Exploratory Study," *Journal of Human Resources* 4(1969):412–436.

12. M. Grossman, "The Correlation Between Health and Schooling."

13. V. R. Fuchs, "Time Preference and Health: An Exploratory Study," in V. R. Fuchs, ed., *Economic Aspects of Health* (Chicago: University of Chicago Press, 1982), pp. 93–120; and A. Bandura, "Self-Efficacy Mechanism in Physiological Activation and Health-Promoting Behavior," in J. Madden IV, ed., *Neural Biology of Learning, Emotion and Affect* (New York: Raven Press, 1991), pp. 229–269.

14. B. C. Vladeck, "Unhealthy Rations," *The American Prospect* (Summer 1991): 102.

15. For other explanations by economic theorists for tied transfers, see N. Bruce and M. Waldman, "Transfers In Kind: Why They Can Be Efficient and Nonpaternalistic," *American Economic Review* 81(1991):1345–1351.

16. See S. Coate, S. Johnson, and R. Zeckhauser, "Robin-Hooding Rents: Exploiting the Pecuniary Effects of In-Kind Programs," (Cambridge, Mass.: Harvard University, March 1992, mimeo).

17. V. R. Fuchs, "From Bismarck to Woodcock: The 'Irrational' Pursuit of National Health Insurance," *Journal of Law and Economics* 19(1976):347–359.

18. V. R. Fuchs, "National Health Insurance Revisited," *Health Affairs* 10(1991):1–11.

19. Personal communication from Ruth Watson Lubic, December 9, 1991.

3

The Politics of Health Care Inequalities

Paul Starr

I take the question "How much inequality in health care can a democratic society tolerate?" as raising, at least by implication, two kinds of problems. The first is historical and empirical: Is there any demonstrable relation between democracy and equality in health care? The second problem is normative and philosophical: How much inequality in health care should democratic principles—and principled democrats—accept?

Either question can refer to the "who" or the "what" of inequality or, as Douglas Rae and his colleagues have put it, the *subjects* or the *domains* of inequality.[1] In regard to the subjects of inequality, we want to know, "Between what different individuals or groups in society do disparities in health care access exist?" The particular subjects of inequality matter for both moral judgment and political analysis. For example, many people would find systematic differences between racial groups in access to health care to be ethically and politically intolerable, while they might be willing to accept equally large differences between random individuals. The correspondence of inequalities in health care to strongly held group identities will also clearly affect the political capacities of the medically underserved and uninsured as well as the response to their claims. Understanding the "who" of inequality requires knowing not only the objective distribution of health services or insurance by income or some other measure, but also what sorts of people, with what identities, resources, numbers, and relations to other groups and institutions, are underserved, uninsured, or otherwise excluded from access to care or protection against its financial risks.

In regard to the domain of inequality, the question is not which people have unequal access but which aspects of health care are differentially accessible. At issue may be access to health services or insurance coverage, entry into health careers, or participation in medical decisionmaking (although here I am concerned only with access to health care and insurance protection). Differences in the domains of inequality, like differences in the subjects, clearly have both moral and political consequences. For example, many people would find unequal access to relatively low-cost, lifesaving medical care to be morally inexcusable but would easily accept equally large differences in access to services that are hugely expensive and merely cosmetic in nature; and they might be at least ambivalent, if not unconcerned, about unequal access to expensive services of unproved effectiveness. Almost inevitably, discussions of the domain of health care inequality invoke or try to define some basic standard of health service or insurance. The standard may variously be conceived as a "decent minimum," the array of services required to satisfy "basic health needs," a standard of "mainstream" care (the care given the middle class), or perhaps a rule of efficacy, cost-effectiveness, or humane respect for an evolving standard of health services financed under a public program.

The task of defining which health benefits or services should be governed by a principle of equality here breaks down into a series of practical and urgent questions of policy: As part of a standard for universal coverage, should we include expensive procedures such as organ transplants that benefit only a few? What about services at the "soft" edge of medical care, such as psychoanalysis, that pose severe problems of moral hazard? What about services over which there are deep moral differences, such as abortion, that threaten political consensus? What about amenities of treatment, such as private hospital rooms, that may affect a patient's sense of propriety or dignity but have no clear effect on the outcome of care? In the terminology I am using, these are questions about *subdomains* of inequality within health care.

Clearly, the analytical complexities are vast and the judgments difficult. But by using the simple distinction between subjects and domains of inequality, we can define a number of politically relevant *inequality situations*. For the purposes of my argument, it will be useful to keep the following situations in mind (which I have deliberately termed *stages* to suggest a kind of hierarchy):

Stage 1: *Mass exclusion from basic coverage*. Under mass exclusion, only a minority in a society have access to health care services and health insurance generally regarded as standard and basic. The majority of the population are, by common definition, underserved and unprotected.

Stage 2: *Minority exclusion from basic coverage*. Under minority exclusion, the mass public has some reasonable level of standard coverage, but a minority of the population still does not.

Where the excluded minority consists of well-defined groups, we can speak of "concentrated minority exclusion." Where the excluded minority consists of diverse and disorganized individuals, we can speak of "dispersed minority exclusion."

Stage 3: *Two- or multitier coverage.* Under a multitier system, the entire population has basic coverage, but some have additional coverage and perhaps privileged access. For example, the wealthy may "opt out" of a public insurance system into a more comprehensive or generous private alternative. A key factor here is the relative size of the upper tier and the base: The politics of a system that is 90 percent public and 10 percent private are profoundly different from the politics of a system that is 90 percent private and 10 percent public. The former we can describe as a system of "broad-based, two-tier coverage"; the latter, as "narrow-based, two-tier coverage."

Stage 4: *Broad-based universalism.* Under a broad-based, universal system, there is essentially one level of coverage for the entire population (although this may or may not mean equally effective access to health care for all segments of society).

Using this simple typology, I come to conclusions that are not entirely happy. Even though I believe mass exclusion from basic coverage is not a stable condition in democratic societies (at least in the economically advanced parts of the world), I see no reason why democratic polities will necessarily be impelled toward broad-based universalism. Under some political conditions, stages two and three seem manageable and stable. Nevertheless, I personally believe that democratic principles should be interpreted as supporting broad-based universalism or at least a broad-based, multitier system. But, as with many things, one must not confuse one's social preferences with historical imperatives.

Democratic Politics and Health Care Inequality

The first of the questions I posed previously—is there is any demonstrable relation between democracy and equality in health care?—invites us to compare democratic and undemocratic societies to see whether the former have more egalitarian distributions of health care. It is by no means obvious that democratic societies do—or why, analytically, they should.

First, the general relation between political democracy and economic equality is ambiguous. Comparative studies of the relation of democracy and inequality—where democracy is defined as regular competitive elections and inequality is usually measured by an index of income inequality, typically the Gini coefficient—come to no firm conclusions. The number of studies that find democracy to be correlated with increased income equality are balanced by those that find no such relation.[2]

Second, although health services and insurance have sometimes been extended more widely as the result of democratically expressed demands, they have also been extended for other reasons, including the interest of undemocratic regimes in legitimating their power. The provision of health care or health insurance is a potent means of promoting goodwill toward the state and encouraging dependence on it. The earliest states in Europe to introduce compulsory health insurance, beginning with Germany, were authoritarian regimes seeking to legitimate themselves in the face of socialist challenges. In our own time, undemocratic socialist regimes, such as Cuba, have used universal health care for the same purpose of legitimation. Regimes also provide public health services out of an interest in creating a healthy work force and a desirable climate for investment and tourism. Democracy need have nothing to do with it.

Third, democratic societies do not allow only the expression of demands for services from those who would otherwise not receive them. They also allow the expression of demands from taxpayers who would prefer not to bear the costs of those services. The question "How much inequality in health care can a democratic society tolerate?" can easily be turned around to read, "How much redistribution of income to provide equality in health care can a democratic society tolerate?" Moreover, in addition to taxpayers, health care providers (particularly physicians) and private industry (particularly insurance companies) have interests that are often at odds with egalitarian state policies. As the *locus classicus* of interest-group politics, health insurance is hardly the place to look for a simple translation of public demands into public policy.

Finally, even though governments of all kinds may provide health care to gain legitimacy, a democratic government might be loath to become liable for all health care services precisely because doing so would unleash demands and provoke conflicts that could prove hard to control. This concern, although not so influential before the 1970s, has since become an increasingly important factor retarding the expansion of public provision.

Taken together, these considerations suggest that political democracy is neither a necessary nor a sufficient condition for universal health insurance or equally accessible health care. Whether there is some general correlation between democracy and health care equality, therefore, seems doubtful, although I know of no comparative, statistical studies measuring the relationship (and I am doubtful, in any event, whether such studies would have a sufficiently reliable and valid base of data to produce useful conclusions).

Yet this is not to say that political democracy has had no effect on the distribution of health care. For even though democracy may not guarantee universalism, it does seem incompatible, as I suggested earlier, with mass exclusion from basic coverage, at least in the economically advanced societies. *That* much inequality does seem to be *too* much inequality to be sustained under a system of majoritarian rule.

To be sure, before the twentieth century universal medical care was not even a demand of democratic movements. The differences in medical treatment received by the rich and the poor did not loom as significant inequalities until a consensus developed that scientific medicine was effective. As belief in medicine grew, so did the economic barriers to care. These were the result of several interrelated changes—professional licensing laws requiring longer training and thereby creating barriers to entry against less expensive practitioners, the development of modern hospitals, and the sheer multiplication of medical services themselves (compare a modern physician fee schedule with its nineteenth-century antecedents). Greater belief in the value of medical care and its higher cost were the conditions under which political pressures increased for state intervention.

These pressures have affected democratic states differently. In some, such as Great Britain and Sweden, the outcome has been broad-based universalism; in others, such as Germany, broad-based, two-tier coverage. In the United States, too, health insurance has expanded, but the development of employee health plans, Medicare, and Medicaid has left roughly one-sixth of the population without insurance coverage. Thus, in the United States the shift during the twentieth century has been from mass to minority exclusion.

That shift can be traced in data on the use of medical services. Just before the impact of the Great Depression, a study by the Committee on the Costs of Medical Care, a privately funded commission, found that use of medical care hinged sharply on family income. (The study did not cover health insurance, which at the time was in its infancy and of no significance in explaining differential access to health care.) In families with less than $1,200 in annual income, 33.5 percent of illnesses received no medical care compared to 7.3 percent of illnesses in families with annual incomes of $10,000 or more. Perhaps most striking for the purposes of this analysis is that in the intervening lower- to middle-income brackets the rates of health care use were more similar to the rates of the poor than to those of the rich. For example, families with $1,200–$1,999 in annual income (35 percent of all families sampled) averaged only 2.27 physician visits per person per year, barely higher than the 2.17 physician visits for families with $1,200 or less annual income (15 percent of families). The rate continued to be relatively flat until the top quarter of the income distribution (more than $3,000), climbing sharply in that group. For the 3.3 percent of families with $10,000 income or more, physician visits averaged 5.32 per person—or more than twice as many as among the poorer half of society.[3] A later study during the Depression suggested that the pattern became even more unequal as families whose incomes dropped from "comfortable" to "poor" cut their use of medical care.[4]

This is the pattern that I have described as mass exclusion: sharply lower use of medical care in the lower-to-middle-income groups compared to the affluent. Like mass poverty more generally, mass exclusion from basic health care disappeared with economic growth after World War II. By 1953, 71 percent of families with incomes between $4,000 and $7, 000 a year had some insurance, compared to 80 percent among those with more income and 41 percent among those with less. Data on the use of medical services indicate sharply diminished differences by family income, although the raw facts need to be interpreted carefully since high use of medical care by the poor partly reflects the concentration among the poor of the aged and the disabled. When adjusted for need, data on health care utilization before and even after 1965 continue to reveal socioeconomic disparities. The pattern, however, differs dramatically from that found by the Committee on the Costs of Medical Care for 1928–1931. Instead of a low, flat curve through the lower half of the income distribution, the curve now tended to climb quickly above the bottom brackets and to flatten out for the upper half. This is the pattern of minority exclusion.[5]

Although by no means the only reason, the major barrier to access by the poor has been the lack of insurance coverage. Why the United States failed to enact a program of universal health insurance during the Progressive Era, the New Deal, and the Truman years is a question I have addressed elsewhere at considerable length.[6] The point worth stressing here is how the pattern of minority exclusion has been sustained for so long. Inadvertently, incremental reform adopted in lieu of national health insurance turned out to be self-limiting, rather than self-extending. The partial, mixed public-private health insurance system that emerged in midcentury, instead of providing the foundations for wider coverage, turned out by the 1970s and 1980s to have become a hindrance to further development. Compromises designed to secure agreement in the passage of Medicare, for example, produced weaknesses in cost control that later made any extension of the federal role appear fiscally irresponsible. The split structure of Medicare and Medicaid—piggybacking the former on Social Security, the latter on welfare—divided the interests of the "worthy" from the "unworthy" poor, reproducing in health care what I have termed elsewhere *the original sin* of U.S. social policy.[7] And the residual uninsured, although numbering more than 30 million, have been a dispersed population unable to organize or articulate any claims on the political system. If the U.S. experience is any indication, political democracy is no protection against dispersed minority exclusion from basic coverage. *That* much inequality is evidently not *too* much inequality for the public conscience to bear—or at least for the political marketplace to ignore.

Today, once again, the issue of universal health insurance is on the political agenda, not so much because of the continuing failure to provide coverage for the excluded, but because of the economic impact of uncontrolled health costs and the increased jeopardy of the middle class. Many people who once thought themselves protected by the employer-provided system are now worried. Many have seen their health coverage erode in recent years as employers have cut and revamped benefits in an effort to hold back costs. With unemployment stalking many families today, Americans fear that when they lose their jobs, they will lose their insurance, and that because of exclusions of preexisting conditions, even if they find a new job with insurance coverage, it may fail to give them full protection. Some small businesses and many of the self-employed find they are being "redlined" as uninsurable. Americans, rather than seeing private insurance expand, as it did in past decades, now face a growing fear of exclusion from coverage—not the exclusion of the poor alone, but the exclusion of risk groups whose members include many middle-class people. And this kind of exclusion may turn out to be the source of far more effective pressure for universal coverage than has yet come from the residual uninsured.[8]

Thus far I have been discussing insurance coverage as if it were tantamount to access to health care. But access to health care is better understood as the product of four sets of variables: the availability of services, the possession of the means of access (money or insurance, transportation), the nondiscriminatory attitudes of health care providers, and the capacities, behavior, and attitudes of the sick themselves, such as their ability to recognize symptoms, communicate with health professionals, and navigate the health care system.

The first two factors have to do with objective resources; the second pair, with subjective attitudes and the abilities of providers and patients. In the early stages of the struggle for health care equality, when reformers are attempting to overcome mass exclusion, objective resources appear to be the entire problem. But with the shift from mass to minority exclusion in the United States, and even under universal systems in other countries, the subjective and behavioral barriers to equality become more prominent. This evolution corresponds to the more general change in the challenges facing social policy with the historic shift from mass poverty to minority poverty in the twentieth century. Substantive equality, it becomes apparent, requires more than formal equality; in health care substantively equal access requires more than equality of insurance coverage. But even though the evidence from other countries suggests that universal health insurance does not eliminate all inequalities of access, it does reduce them, and it particularly reduces the likelihood that sickness will be impoverishing. As a basis of criticism, a perfectionist standard can be useful; but if misunderstood, it can undermine efforts to achieve equal insurance protection. In health care, as in life, the best should not be the enemy of the good.

Democratic Principles and Health Care Inequality

I turn now to the second question: How much inequality in health care should democratic principles—and principled democrats—accept? Throughout the Western democracies, the idea of governmental action to ensure universal health insurance is no longer controversial. One recent survey of the United States, Great Britain, France, Canada, and West Germany showed the overwhelming majorities in all five countries agreeing with the statements "Nobody, however sick and however poor, should be bankrupted by paying for the cost of their medical care," and "People who are unemployed and poor should be able to get the same amount and quality of medical services as people who have good jobs and are paying substantial taxes."[9] This survey suggests that public values about health care inequality are not nearly as disparate as the actual practices and institutions in the five societies.

In the United States, the exclusion of one of six citizens from basic health coverage has few defenders. Almost all seem to recognize that minority exclusion is wrong and that some governmental action to rectify that situation is in principle justifiable. Since no corrective action has in fact been taken, this may seem no more than hypocrisy, but it is significant. Those who are not generally egalitarians now seem to accept what James Tobin once described as "specific egalitarianism"—that is, an ideal of equality restricted to a particular domain of social life, such as health care. Health care, liberals and most conservatives in democratic societies agree, is "special"—not to be treated like an ordinary commodity on the market because of the distinctive needs of the sick or their vulnerabilities or because of the peculiar, endemic failures of unregulated insurance markets.[10] Even those, such as Alain Enthoven, who favor market-based measures typically call for them now as a mechanism, not for allocating insurance only to those able to pay, but for promoting cost-conscious consumer choice of health plans.[11]

Yet while hardly anyone disagrees that everyone should have health insurance, there continue to be deep and wide disagreements in the United States about the policies needed to bring about that result. Some of this disagreement is practical: How do we get from here to there? But some disagreement also concerns exactly where *there* should be: How far do democratic principles obligate us to go in the direction of equality? In the terminology I have been using, much of this debate can be described as a split between those who find multitier coverage acceptable and those who believe that democratic principles require nothing less than broad-based universalism.

Philosophically, the split between the two involves two different conceptions of what democratic ideals require in health care. On the one hand, the defenders of multitier coverage see the objective of reform as raising the poor and the uninsured to what might be described as a standard of adequate protection. Some see that standard as only a decent minimum; others define it more liberally as the standard of mainstream care. In a system of multitier coverage, people who want to purchase a higher level of insurance or privileged treatment can do so. On the other hand, the advocates of broad-based universalism see the objective as equal health care for all, which means creating a uniform system that treats rich and poor alike. In the universalists' view, getting the rich to ride in the same boat as the poor and the middle class is the best insurance of all. ("Have you ever noticed," a medical journalist once said to me, "that most people who call for two-tier systems expect to be in the upper tier?")

In practice, the split between these two currents of thinking revolves around several key issues. First, the advocates of universalism tend to favor a single, public health insurance system (as in Canada) or a national health service (as in Great Britain), whereas the advocates of multitier coverage want more diversity, pluralism, and competition. Second, the defenders of universalism generally want the sphere of universal coverage to be defined in comprehensive terms to embrace virtually all health care services, whereas the advocates of multitier coverage are more willing to accept limitations on the scope of public (or publicly mandated) coverage, thereby leaving more room for variable (hence unequal), supplementary insurance. Third, the advocates of universalism often want actively to discourage development of private alternatives to public financing on the grounds that any use of the market mechanism tends to reproduce and widen inequalities. The defenders of multitier coverage are less disturbed by such inequalities as long as everyone has adequate protection for basic health needs.

In a sense, the split I am describing is the classic division between social democracy and liberal democracy. But health care is a peculiar case in that debate, if only because the social democratic alternative in health care, exemplified by Britain and Canada, has turned out to absorb fewer resources and, in particular, to have lower administrative costs—the rare case where more equality, less spending, and less bureaucracy come together. The general liberal preference for pluralism and competition also runs up against the reality in health care that competitive insurance plans tend to seek out the most favorable health risks rather than produce health care more efficiently.[12] Thus, many people who generally favor the liberal democratic preference for decentralized market mechanisms switch sides when it comes to health care—one instance where social democracy seems to be more fiscally responsible as well as more equitable.

Yet even those who prefer broadly based universalism in health care, as I do, must acknowledge the huge political obstacles to adopting it in the United States. Is there any compromise short of universalism, then, that could be acceptable? The intermediate position that I earlier described as broad-based, multitier coverage does offer such a possibility.

The chief danger of a two-tier system is the segregation of the poor in a lower tier, or base, that over time becomes distinctly inferior, even if not intended to be. The deterioration is far more likely if the base is narrow, chiefly serving the poor. In that case, middle-class voters will resent paying taxes to support the base, and they will tend to insist that the public sector offer no more than a decent minimum. If, however, middle-class voters get their own health insurance through the public system, they will be more generous in their views on the appropriate level of fiscal support and probably not begrudge the poor equal terms of access to that system. Thus, broad-based, multitier coverage is likely to generate a mainstream, middle-class standard of care for a majority of society that includes the poor.

This is the pattern of the German health insurance system, where nine out of ten people are covered by the publicly regulated sickness funds and only one of nine by commercial insurance. The balance is partly maintained by a rule that the decision to opt out of the sickness funds is an irreversible lifetime decision: Once someone buys commercial insurance, they lose eligibility for the sickness funds.

The German insurance system does not eliminate inequalities at the top, but it does minimize inequalities at the bottom. And this seems to me to satisfy the key democratic interests in health care—the inclusion of the poor in a mainstream standard of care and their protection against impoverishment from sickness. Admittedly, such a system fails to achieve perfect equality of treatment since it does not prevent the rich from using their wealth to get privileged attention. But to insist on equal treatment at the top as well as at the bottom is to pursue a course that is likely to generate more opposition to egalitarian health policies, and more interference in private choice, than is necessary or wise. To be treated as an equal in a democratic society does not mean that we must be equal in all our possessions and facets of life, but rather that we enjoy a fundamental equality of respect and dignity. And in health care that respect and dignity can be assured without imposing a uniform standard on the affluent as long as the standard of care for the poor is no different from the standard available to the majority.

Summary

Let me see if I can pull together the threads of the preceding argument. In answer to the question "How much inequality in health care can a democratic society tolerate?" I have given two answers. First, from a historical perspective, mass exclusion clearly has been too much inequality for democratic societies to accept, but, as the U.S. case illustrates, democracy does not immunize a society against minority exclusion from basic coverage and equal access. Second, democratic principles, at least as I understand them, argue not only against minority exclusion but also against what I have described as narrow-based, multitier coverage. Yet broad-based universalism should not be regarded as the only acceptable answer. By minimizing inequalities at the bottom, even if allowing for privileges at the top, broad-based, multitier coverage seems to me to achieve the chief democratic interests.

Notes

1. D. Rae et al., *Inequalities* (Cambridge, Mass.: Harvard University Press, 1981).

2. L. Sirowy and A. Inkeles, "The Effects of Democracy on Economic Growth and Inequality: A Review," in A. Inkeles, ed., *On Measuring Democracy: Its Consequences and Concomitants* (New Brunswick, N.J.: Transaction, 1991), pp. 125–156.

3. I. S. Falk et al., *The Incidence of Illness and the Receipt and Costs of Medical Care Among Representative Families* (Chicago: University of Chicago Press, 1932), pp. 103, 281, 283.

4. G. St. Perrot, E. Sydenstricker, and S. D. Collins, "Medical Care During the Depression," *Milbank Memorial Fund Quarterly* 12(April 1934):99–114.

5. For a more extended discussion of the data and the transition from mass to minority exclusion (which I formerly termed *mass inequality* and *marginal inequality*), see P. Starr, "Medical Care and the Pursuit of Equality in America," in President's Commission for the Study of Ethical Problems in Medicine and Biomedical and Behavioral Research, *Securing Access to Health Care* (Washington, D.C.: Government Printing Office, March 1983), vol. 2, Appendices, 2–22.

6. P. Starr, *The Social Transformation of American Medicine* (New York: Basic Books, 1982), Book 2, Chapter 1.

7. P. Starr, "Health Care for the Poor: The Past Twenty Years," in S. Danziger and D. Weinberg, eds., *Fighting Poverty: What Works and What Doesn't* (Cambridge, Mass.: Harvard University Press, 1986), pp. 106–132.

8. For a more extended discussion of these issues, see P. Starr, "The Middle Class and National Health Reform," *The American Prospect* 6(Summer 1991):7–12.

9. H. Taylor and U. E. Reinhardt, "Does the System Fit?" *Health Management Quarterly* 12(1991):2–10.

10. On the "specialness" of health care, see N. Daniels, *Just Health Care* (Cambridge: Cambridge University Press, 1985); and K. J. Arrow, "Uncertainty and the Welfare Economics of Medical Care," *American Economic Review* 53(Dececember 1963):941–968.

11. A. C. Enthoven, *Health Plan: The Only Practical Solution to the Soaring Cost of Medical Care* (Reading, Mass.: Addison-Wesley, 1980); and A. C. Enthoven, "Managed Competition: An Agenda for Action," *Health Affairs* (Summer 1988):25–47.

12. On the limitations of Enthoven's competitive model, see S. B. Jones, "Can Multiple Choice Be Managed to Constrain Health Care Costs?" *Health Affairs* (Fall 1989):51–59.

4

Poverty, Public Health, and Tuberculosis Control in New York City: Lessons from the Past

Margaret A. Hamburg

Poverty is a public health issue. Too many recent reports and studies have documented the poor health status of minority and low-socioeconomic populations, and sadly some of the grossest disparities in health and health indicators are cited from New York City.

With more than a quarter of all New Yorkers—some 1.3 million people—without health insurance, some 60 percent of the city's children living in families below or near the poverty level, and enormous gaps in primary care and other health care providers in the poorest communities, it is evident that poverty and inadequate access to medical services must underlie many of the distressingly high rates of serious disease, disability, and death we face.

Infectious diseases such as tuberculosis, HIV infection/AIDS, syphilis, and measles have been on the rise. Correspondingly, many New York communities are plagued by rates of substance abuse, violence, and infant mortality that far outstrip the national average.

I could give you a long list of statistics, but the point is simple: The problems are severe and worsening. And in many cases, even though we have the medical knowledge and technology to prevent and control disease, we are failing in our efforts to apply that know-how to the health of all our citizenry.

Traditionally, local agencies have sought to be the provider of last resort. Yet the harsh realities of the discrepancy between the magnitude of the need and the resources of urban health departments, such as New York City's, are overwhelming. Tuberculosis—a disease known to be intimately linked to poverty—is one case in point.

We now hear with almost daily regularity that TB is back with a vengeance in New York City, and the numbers are alarming. In 1990, there were more than 3, 500 cases reported—a 38 percent increase over the previous year—and preliminary data indicate an even higher case count for 1991.

New York City's overall TB incidence rate, roughly 50 per 100,000, is more than five times the national rate and more than three times the rate considered epidemic by the Centers for Disease Control. All told, the city accounts for 15 percent of the nation's caseload. But citywide figures tend to obscure the disproportionate manner in which TB targets the poor.

That TB remains intertwined with poverty is beyond doubt. The health districts with the highest case rates—Central Harlem (with a case rate more than three times that of the city), the Lower East Side, East Harlem, Morrissania, Bedford, Bushwick, Fort Greene, and Mott Haven—are among the city's poorest.

And because these areas of concentrated inner-city poverty are overwhelmingly communities of color, the disproportionate burden of illness on racial and ethnic minority groups is dramatic. New TB cases are occurring thirteen times more frequently among African Americans than among whites; the incidence rate among African American men aged 25 to 44—the hardest hit of any group in the city—is estimated at twenty times higher than among white men in that age group.

Other indicators of poverty and deteriorating social conditions are also evident in the profile of those at risk for TB. The homeless and those with unstable housing are disproportionately represented among TB cases—one recent study done at a large public hospital in New York City suggested a figure close to 70 percent. Many are in, out, and unfortunately back in the city's correction system. High rates of alcohol and drug use (both intravenous and crack) are also found among TB cases. In addition, a disproportionately large number of new TB cases are associated with HIV disease—a disease that, of course, cuts across all socioeconomic levels but is increasingly concentated in poor and minority communities.

What is the current state of TB control in New York City? In a recent article, Karen Brudney and Jay Dobkin describe in graphic and alarming detail some of the current problems.[1] Their study of a prospective cohort of 224 patients of TB admitted to Harlem Hospital during 1988 revealed that 89 percent of those diagnosed and discharged failed to complete treatment and that 27 percent were readmitted with active TB within twelve months. More specifically, more than 50 percent of the TB patients discharged received no follow-up treatment, more than 25 percent were lost to follow-up within three months, and another 10 percent were lost to follow-up after the three-month point. In sum, close to nine out of ten did not complete the full course of therapy they required.

Not surprisingly, within a year of discharge more than one-quarter of these patients were readmitted at least once with confirmed active TB, and almost all of these patients were again lost to follow-up. Within seven months of the cutoff date for the sampling, one-fifth of the originally discharged TB patients had been readmitted yet a third time with active TB.

The problem of noncompliance or failure to successfully complete a full course of therapy was significantly associated with homelessness and alcoholism. Crack users were totally noncompliant in the study. People with HIV symptoms were more likely to be compliant than asymptomatic HIV-infected TB patients.

These numbers are bleak. Clearly many factors have come together to fuel the epidemic of TB we now face—the overlapping epidemics of poverty, homelessness, substance abuse, and HIV. But budget cuts and the lack of serious and ongoing commitment to maintaining basic public health services and infrastructure—particulary in our most underprivileged communities—clearly paved the way for much of what we are currently scrambling to control.

Now that we are well into a period of intense budgetary constraint, the New York City Health Department and the many other entities that struggle to provide health care to the poor are continually grappling with the problem of how to maintain services and respond to new health needs, all the while holding the line against further erosion of the meager resources with which we do our work. I cannot minimize how difficult that struggle is. But the resurgence of TB is a powerful reminder of what will happen when we do not hold the line—when we allow living conditions for low-income and minority populations to deteriorate and allow budget pressures to strip away vital public health functions.

I want to briefly discuss the history of tuberculosis control in New York City—not in the early days of TB before the advent of understanding of the disease's cause and mode of transmission allowed sound prevention measures to be initiated or before the advent of antibiotics enabled treatment and cure. Rather, I wish to examine events beginning not more than 15 or so years ago, when we had the tools to control this disease, but—as the growing caseload now attests—despite being one of the most medically and technologically advanced cities on earth, we failed a fundamental mission of public health.

Tuberculosis is now the subject of considerable attention not only in the city but also at the state and federal level. Not only is the disease resurgent; it is also more pernicious than it was in the past because of multiple drug resistance and because of the existence of a huge reservoir of immune-deficient and otherwise susceptible persons—often located in crowded congregate settings such as jails and shelters—who lie directly in the path of TB transmission.

But as we grapple with the failure that led to epidemic TB in 1992, we must look beyond blaming it on the emergence of HIV, although most of the recent attention has focused on the role of AIDS as the underlying cause. For although there is evidence that HIV has "primed the pump" of TB disease, a broad view of the social conditions that spawn TB seems to indicate that an increase in TB incidence would have occurred even without the appearance of HIV.

Let me quote briefly from a Health Department document:

> It will become quite apparent to anyone who reads this ... that the disease thought by many to be disappearing is still very much with us. You will note that a[n] ... increase in newly reported cases has been documented. ... You will also observe that tuberculosis has been diagnosed among the younger population and in particular in young children under the age of four. Cases occurring among the young [are] evidence that tuberculosis is being actively transmitted in our city and [dispel] the theory that tuberculosis is disappearing as a public health problem. The existence of extensive knowledge on tuberculosis makes it a controllable and eradicable disease, but because of funding shortages and inadequate resources, tuberculosis remains a serious public health problem in our city. A new interest and dedication regarding tuberculosis [have] emerged during [the year]. It is hoped that if a consistent and sustained control effort can be maintained through [the next decade], transmission will be prevented, case rates will decrease and tuberculosis can in a practical sense be eradicated.[2]

The year was 1979, and the coming decade—during which, it was hoped, TB could be practically eradicated—was the 1980s. The document cited was the Health Department's 1979 annual TB report.

Sadly, the 1979 report marked the first year that cases began to increase after *decades* of steady decline. But it should be noted that even when TB was at its nadir in New York City, it was allowed to linger, and even fester, in impoverished neighborhoods such as Central Harlem—where the incidence rate was three times the city average and four times the national average—the Lower East Side, and Fort Greene, communities that have long been plagued by poverty, unemployment, poor access to health care, substandard housing, and homelessness.

And even though HIV was, unbeknownst to us, already in our midst, it is unlikely that the number of HIV-infected had yet sufficiently mushroomed or that there would have been enough HIV-infected persons far along into the disease process for HIV to have been a significant cause of the initial upswing in TB in the late 1970s.

Just what did reverse the trend of decreasing TB? Some telling and cogent analysis has already been done to answer this question. It is striking that the rise in TB in the late 1970s reflected drastic cuts in the Health Department's TB Control Program in the immediately preceding period. What transpired should be a cautionary tale.

In 1968, the TB program had a $40 million budget, which supported 22 chest clinics, another 6 clinics run jointly with the city hospitals, and more than 1,000 designated TB hospital beds. Also in 1968, a TB task force appointed by Mayor John Lindsay recommended that the TB beds be phased out at the rate of 100 per year and that they be replaced by an expanded integrated community outreach and control program for TB patients.

Basically, this made sense. With the advent of better oral drugs, long-term inpatient care seemed unnecessarily expensive, and ambulatory care became a feasible way to treat patients. An outpatient system could certainly be created to cater to the special needs of TB patients and ensure compliance.

It was explicitly stated at that time that money saved from the closing of the TB beds would be used to create a sophisticated outpatient program and that methadone programs would be linked up to the health department and become involved in treating methadone patients with TB. In addition, clinics would operate in the evenings and possibly Saturdays, and home visits would be made regularly to enhance compliance. Finally, long-term domiciliary care would be available for homeless patients with TB. Recommended funding for the outreach effort was set at $18 million per year by 1973.

What happened? Ten years later the beds were gone, but combined city-state funding for the outpatient program totaled less than $2 million. In the mid-1970s, New York City's fiscal crisis led to enormous cuts in the monies for all public health programs, including TB. At the same time, New York state cut back and then terminated its support for the city's TB control activities. The state had provided half of such funding just a few years earlier.

Similarly, the federal contribution decreased 80 percent, from nearly $1.5 million in 1974 to a little more than $250,000 by 1980. In 1978, the city's yearly TB spending was down to about $24 million, well below the $40 million yearly of a decade earlier, and the bulk of funding now went to inpatient costs, which were on the decline. Only $1.6 million was devoted to TB control activities, and only nine of 22 chest clinics remained.

In 1980, after the city's TB rate had begun to increase for the first time in decades, another TB task force, this one empaneled by the Council of Lung Associations of New York, decried what it called the "fiscal neglect" of TB control activities and the "failure of both health authorities and government at all levels to muster a public health program." That same year, a federally supported pilot project targeting patients at high risk of treatment failure was begun. The Supervised Therapy Program, as it was called, proved enormously successful. But no branch of government would enable the program to expand beyond the pilot level, and Supervised Therapy still consisted of only a half dozen or so workers in 1989. Throughout the 1980s, there were no significant increases in TB support despite the accelerating incidence rate.

Currently, the Health Department has some $11.3 million with which to control resurgent TB—in the context of HIV, increased homelessness, economic downturn, and multiple drug resistance. The federal government's allotment in this crucial endeavor amounts to some $3.5 million, which seems meager in view of the Department of Health and Human Services's stated goal of TB eradication by the year 2010.

Lee Reichman has added yet another layer of context to the sad state of recent TB control history in New York. There is a ubiquitous occurrence in public health practice, states Reichman, called "the U-shaped curve of concern."[3] If we graph the city's (or the nation's) TB rate over time, we will see the uncanny resemblance between that graph and the letter U. The first half of the U represents the drop-off in cases effected through collective public health efforts. Then resources for disease control are withdrawn because of success and the inability of public health leadership to further demonstrate "compelling need." Predictably, incidence of the once-controlled disease again rises in proportion to the removal of resources—thus, the second half of the U.

We are all now just beginning to find out how costly, in terms of human suffering *and* economics, the second half of that U can be with regard to tuberculosis. The lesson is rendered all the more painful by the knowledge that not only did society choose to pass on the relatively inexpensive option available to it, but also that those of us in public health *let* it slide.

If we *have* learned our lesson, what might we be anticipating as we steel ourselves for the upcoming rounds in the battle against TB? And, moreover, how do we most effectively fight TB in the context of the larger public health crisis that is already upon us?

I think we must begin by factoring into all of our efforts the recognition that poverty is the ultimate driving force behind the spread of TB. Just as we cannot expect to cure poverty, neither can we expect to treat TB solely with a few spoonfuls of medicine.

In the case of poverty-linked TB, we therefore need to understand—and to make those whose support we *need* understand—what it is we must do if we want homeless, HIV-infected, substance-abusing, and otherwise troubled New Yorkers to complete their treatment regimens. If we expect to succeed in bringing TB under control and in beating back the specter of multi-drug-resistant strains refractory to our best treatment efforts, we had better ensure the appropriate and complete course of therapy for all with TB disease. To do so, we must have:

- Effective and accessible clinics where active cases get first priority
- Accountable outreach programs and a large cadre of trained, motivated workers to administer directly observed therapy to outpatients
- Positive incentive programs—using free meals, carfare, or even cash—in exchange for supervised treatment
- Information—procured through pilot programs and the like—about which incentives work (we must then *use* them extensively because incentives are ultimately cheaper than treatment failure)

We will also need to develop a range of live-in facilities, with appropriate levels of care, where people with TB who do not require acute hospitalization but do need considerable support—often including housing or some level of medical care or both—can reside while they are receiving their full course of therapy or for as long as they need that enhanced level of support. In that regard, we will need to look at increasing the capacity of special shelters with enhanced services for homeless persons with TB—there is currently only one 85-bed shelter of this type for men in the city and *not one bed* for women.

In a small minority of cases, some individuals may be required to complete their treatment course, either through mandatory supervised therapy or confinement until cure is achieved. Clearly any form of long-term detention must be an infrequently used last resort—an extreme remedy for cases where all efforts to engage the individual in ongoing treatment have repeatedly failed, with documented disease relapses and documented refusal to comply with appropriate therapy. Due process, an appearance before a judge, and every effort to protect civil liberties must be an integral component of any such treatment mechanism.

In addition, we must institute aggressive measures to stop the institutional spread of TB: in hospitals, shelters, prisons, drug treatment centers, and so on. We must have adequate medical facilities to ensure appropriate respiratory isolation and infection control during the infectious stages of disease and appropriate environmental conditions/housing arrangements to reduce risk of transmission to both staff and client population. We must screen, case-find, and undertake preventive therapy—focusing first on the most high-risk populations and settings. We must improve the quality of medical care for TB patients, including staff and provider education and training to ensure appropriate diagnosis and treatment, as well as improve the quality and timing of laboratory functions. We must improve research and development in the TB arena to enhance our efforts at

TB prevention, diagnosis and control. We must educate the public about this disease. Finally, we must advocate for more resources to fulfill these missions.

If we are to succeed in our efforts to prevent and control TB, we had better not hedge in implementing these required steps—we know what to do and have known what to do for years. Nevertheless, we do have to ask and answer many questions, particularly in an era of limited resources. For example, how can we most effectively target interventions and establish priorities among competing needs? How can we foster public-private partnerships? What new, innovative, and perhaps nontraditional methodologies might be adopted in an effort to get a near-impossible job done? What long-term ramifications might spring from the reestablishment of single-disease institutions?

It is also appropriate that we draw attention to the increasingly intractable nature of the health crises that confront, and even batter, public health departments, crises that have everything to do with poverty but end up primarily on our doorstep because they manifest as disease processes.

Control of tuberculosis in New York City is entirely possible. The disease itself, with few exceptions, is still curable, and the cost of the medications is still relatively inexpensive. Access to health care, directly observed therapy, and positive incentives are all attainable goals.

To achieve these goals, resources will be required. Yet however large the monetary investment in TB control may be, it does not compare with the financial costs that we will face later if we fail to take decisive action now. Each new case costs the city between $15,000 and $250,000 in treatment and related expenses—more for the difficult to manage, relapsing cases and for cases of multiple-drug-resistant TB.

It is painfully clear that we now need to spend significantly greater amounts of money to subdue a disease that we could have controlled if adequate resources had been allocated five, ten, 15, or 20 years ago. Correspondingly, the future cost of failing to aggressively address this resurgent problem now will be prohibitive.

Unfortunately, tuberculosis is not the only preventable disease on the rise in New York City and other urban areas thanks to the legacy of neglect, cutbacks in public health, and reductions in programs to provide critical health services. Further cutbacks in public health will ensure that these epidemics of disease extend into the next decade, and we will pay both with the future health of our citizens and with higher health care costs for treating the victims of preventable diseases.

Solutions will not come easily. Clearly they will require political determination, massive mobilization, creativity, and unprecedented coordination of energy and resources at all levels. At a very minimum, we should learn from the past.

Notes

1. K. Brudney and J. Dobkin, "Resurgent Tuberculosis in New York City," *American Review of Respiratory Diseases* 144(1991):745–749.

2. New York City Department of Health, *Annual Tuberculosis Report* (1979).

3. L. Reichman, "The U-Shaped Curve of Concern," *American Review of Respiratory Diseases* 144(1991):741–742.

5

Inequalities in Health

Douglas Black

It is part of the conventional wisdom that socioeconomic deprivation is associated with demonstrable "ill-health" in affected individuals and groups, such ill-health being manifested in high levels of morbidity and, perhaps most convincingly, in high levels of mortality. And it is also part of conventional social idealism, expressed in the declaration of Alma Ata and accepted with enthusiasm by both the central office of the World Health Organization in Geneva and its regional branches, that an important objective in the health field is to reduce these socially related inequalities in health experience. This particular aspiration is sometimes given misplaced concreteness by such phrases as "to reduce inequalities in health by a quarter by the year 2000."

It is certainly not my purpose in this chapter to question the facts that have virtually established an association between social deprivation and ill-health. On the contrary, I hope to demonstrate them at least in outline, for they are now overwhelming. Still less do I wish to disparage the idealism that says, "Here is an evil. What can we do about it?" But the central thesis of my chapter is that progress in this important matter has to be based on detailed analysis and that at least in those countries that are privileged to call themselves "developed," it is more likely to be achieved by what Popper calls "piecemeal social engineering" (including some medical measures) than by some utopian recasting of society designed to abolish poverty and its consequences at a stroke.[1] This attitude may be criticized for lack of vision, but years of medical practice tend to induce a bias toward pragmatism over a blind faith in the sweeps and surges of political upheaval.

My initial involvement with this problem was almost a matter of chance. A career in academic internal medicine had led me along devious paths to a post, curiously designated that of "chief scientist," in the U.K. Department of Health and Social Security. My prime duty lay in the administration of research commissioned by the department; but like any other civil servant, I was subject to instruction from the current secretary of state. At that time, the post was held by David Ennals, who was unusual among politicians in having worked in the health field and in having discharged his responsibilities on their merits, not as a means of personal political advancement. At any rate, one day in 1977 I was called to his office and asked to bring together a working group to examine the relationship between social class and health. Even an unusual politician is still a politician, and he may have hoped the study might reveal links of such a nature that they could be corrected by a few simple and inexpensive measures within the health services. From such a "quick fix," the reality was to prove somewhat different, but I am partisan enough to ascribe to our efforts a different kind of value, that of stimulating others to tackle with improved methodology a problem that, though well recognized in outline, had not been subjected to multidisciplinary examination on the basis of comprehensive health statistics.

DHSS Working Group on Inequalities in Health (1977–1980)

A working group that produces a report that is still quoted after more than a decade must be considered to have justified its name, if not all the expectations that may have been placed on it. Other members of the group might have a different perspective, but the factors to which I ascribe the success of the group are these:

1. It was small, with only four members including the chair. This size required that members be chosen only as potential contributors, not as representatives of organizations.
2. It was balanced in discipline, with two doctors and two sociologists. Of the doctors, one was a clinician (myself), the other a public health doctor (J. N. Morris, epidemiologist). Of the sociologists, one was "radical" (Peter Townsend, then of Essex, now of Bristol), the other "conservative" (Cyril Smith, secretary of the Social Science Research Council).
3. It met often enough—about once a month—for momentum to be sustained.
4. It had excellent fact-finding backup both from two research assistants, Stuart Blume and Nicky Hart, and from the resources of a sizable government department.
5. It was left alone to do its work not only by the Labour administration that set it up, but also by the Conservative administration that took over—although the later reception of the report suggests the Conser-

> vatives may not have entirely foreseen what they were about to receive, nor were they particularly thankful.

I confess that I cannot now recall whether we were given terms of reference or were asked to write our own. But the broad objectives we are said to have been given are on the record as follows:[2]

- To assemble available information about the differences in health status among the social classes and about contributory factors, including relevant data from other industrial countries
- To analyze this material for the purpose of identifying possible causal relationships, to examine and then test the hypotheses, and to assess the implications for policy
- To suggest what further research might be initiated

Information on Deprivation and Health Status

In place of the phrase "among the social classes" in the first of our objectives, I have used "deprivation." The formal reason for this substitution is that there is no way of ascribing social class to individuals in census data since what is recorded is the occupation of individuals. A more substantial reason is the likelihood that social or even occupational status is not a direct determinant of health experience but is a crude reflection of socioeconomic advantage or disadvantage. Although affluence has an influence on health, its effects are trivial compared with those of deprivation—when subjected to statistical inquiry, the "diseases of affluence" prove somewhat elusive.

In essence, we were being asked to compare quantitatively socioeconomic status and health experience. We discovered, however, that existing measures suffered from considerable inadequacies. One of the most important aspects of our report was to draw attention to these and so to stimulate the development of more satisfactory indices, some of which will be mentioned later.

Assessment of Socioeconomic Status

In the absence of direct information on the social class of individuals in Britain, we used the extensive information on the occupation of individuals obtained in the census carried out at ten-year intervals—the Decennial Census of the Office of Populations, Censuses, and Surveys (OPCS). Occupations are divided into six broad groups as follows:

1. Professional, such as accountant, doctor, or lawyer (6 percent)
2. Intermediate, such as nurse or schoolteacher (23 percent)

3. Skilled nonmanual, such as secretary or shop assistant (12 percent)
4. Skilled manual, such as bus driver or carpenter (36 percent)
5. Partly skilled, such as postal worker or bus conductor (17 percent)
6. Unskilled, such as laborer or cleaner (6 percent)

The percentages ascribed to these categories are of the total number of economically active and retired males at the time of the 1981 census. These categories at once highlight two major limitations of current the data: the lack of adequate occupational information on women and on the unemployed. The assumption that wives are adequately characterized in that respect by the occupation of their husbands is increasingly unsound as more wives go out to work, in some cases in occupations "superior" in status to that of their husbands. When a man becomes unemployed, he is not separately categorized but is allocated to his previous occupation. Although no class of occupation is immune, the risk of unemployment is higher in manual than in nonmanual occupations. Since unemployment is itself a cause of mental and physical ill-health, its nonrandom distribution will add to any apparent health disadvantage of manual occupations; conversely, measures that effectively diminish unemployment can be expected to advantage manual workers disproportionally.

Even these limited number of examples indicate that the allocation of specific occupations to these categories is to some extent arbitrary; and indeed minor reallocations of occupations take place between one census and the next, something that becomes relevant when the relation between occupational status and health is to be studied over time. The overall effect of this allocation is, however, small in comparison with a true change in the proportion of people employed in the broad categories of occupation, more people being employed in professional and similar occupations and fewer in unskilled manual occupations. For example, in the 50 years between 1931 and 1981 the percentage of economically active men in occupational classes I and II (professional and intermediate) rose from 14 to 29, while the percentage in classes IV and V (semiskilled and unskilled manual) fell from 38 to 23. By comparison, there was no numerical change in class III (skilled nonmanual and manual). This surely implies that whatever benefits to health may accrue from following a professional type of occupation are now more widely distributed and that the health disadvantages of manual work now affect a smaller proportion of the population. There is no cause for complacency, however, for the health disadvantages still affect millions of people and are no less intense for the affected individual than they ever were.

As against these limitations, the OPCS data have two great advantages. They cover the entire population of some 50 million in England and Wales, and they can be related to strict measures of mortality and to somewhat looser measures of morbidity. The very large numbers in the occupational subgroups confer statistical robustness on the findings, a claim supported by consistent findings in the United Kingdom a decade later and by comparable findings in other industrial countries.[3] The linkage of occupational data obtained by a census to mortality data in occupational groups involves a time lag—the moment of completing a census form is seldom the moment of death. This difficulty, inherent in any cross-sectional study, can be radically resolved only by long-term longitudinal studies, such as are now in process.[4] But at least the data we used for mortality and morbidity were on the same nationwide basis and were carried out by the same organization, the OPCS.

Before leaving the assessment of socioeconomic status to discuss our measures of mortality and morbidity in some detail, I wish to note some later developments. These stem in part at least from a realization that even though occupation is in many ways a suitable, readily obtained indicator of affluence or deprivation, it is also a rather crude one because of the variations in economic status among people who are ostensibly members of the same trade or profession. Income or salary would be a more direct economic indicator, but there are obvious difficulties of validation and confidentiality. An important trend has been to move away from unitary measures of socioeconomic status, such as occupation or income, to indices that take account of discrete aspects of lifestyle associated with the level of available resources. Components of such indices include the number of persons per room in a house, car ownership, unemployment, single parenthood, owned or rented house tenure, and receipt of means-tested benefits. This type of information may not be readily obtainable nationally, but it can be sought in specific surveys of different areas in a conurbation and linked with the health statistics for the same areas. Such detailed surveys may not only be a check on the validity of results obtained from less detailed national surveys but may also allow separate analysis of the discrete component factors in deprivation.

Assessment of Health Status

It is a sad fact that the most generally available and most reliable indicator of health status should be the likelihood of death, whether expressed as a mortality rate or as life expectancy. In Britain, death certificates are transmitted to the OPCS, which in due course issues reports on mortality by occupation. We used the 1978 OPCS report, the latest available at the time of compiling our own report. A death certificate is at least reliable evidence of the fact of death, even if the certified cause of death may include an element of speculation. I believe we were right to derive our main evidence from what turned out to be gross differences in mortality according to occupation, without prejudice to realizing that there is more to quality of life than the likelihood of early death.

Our chief source of information on the state of health of the living was the General Household Survey carried out by the OPCS. Since 1971, a sample of 15, 000 households have been asked annually about housing, including tenure of occupancy; occupation and whether currently employed; education; and mobility. This information is then available for comparison with information on state of health collected at the same time. The subjects of the survey are asked about both acute illness and chronic illness or disability. This type of self-reported information on health lacks diagnostic precision but is adequate to outline the general pattern of the relationship between occupational status and health. Information on how occupational status affects specific types of disease can be obtained nationally from death certificates; and the pattern of illness experienced during life can be deduced from the collected records of selected general practices collated under the auspices of the Royal College of General Practitioners.

Since our report was published in 1980, there have been important developments in methods for assessing health status. More detailed information on smaller groups is being gathered and includes data on social factors, including occupation, as well as other aspects of economic status. There has also been a shift of emphasis away from preoccupation with tangible diseases toward greater concern with how people feel and how well they function both at work and in leisure pursuits—in other words, with quality of life. There are now a number of validated procedures for assessing quality of life, some designed to be completed by a physician or social worker and others intended to be self-administered. The domains of well-being (or ill-being) that need to be explored are the psychological (how people feel about themselves), the physical (organic disability), the occupational (fitness for and at work), and the social (personal relations and leisure activities). The methodology for assessing quality of life in the healthy and in the victims of specific states of disease (e.g., tumors, arthritis, AIDS, terminal illness) has been comprehensively and critically assessed.[5]

Deprivation and Health

It was already well recognized even before we began our study that among the disadvantages of poverty must be included substantial ill-health. Our factual contribution was to quantitate the relationship on a broad basis of national statistics. Our findings have been reported in some detail,[6] and I need only illustrate them here. Table 5.1 sets out the death rates per 1,000 per annum for men and women between the ages of 15 and

TABLE 5.1
Death Rates per 1,000 People per Year, 1971

Class		Men	Women
I		3.98	2.15
II		5.54	2.85
III	(nonmanual)	5.80	2.76
III	(manual)	6.08	3.41
IV		7.00	4.27
V		9.88	5.31

64 in the occupational classes I to V in England and Wales in 1971. Not only is there a striking difference between the extremes; there is also a relatively steady gradation of disadvantage in respect of death rate from one occupational group to the next in both sexes. This gradation strengthens the likelihood that we are exposing a real phenomenon, not just meeting a statistical artifact at the extremes of a range. The higher death rate of manual as compared with nonmanual workers during their working life is not only shared with their wives, as shown in the table; it is also experienced by their children, and it follows them into old age.

Other sensitive indicators of poor health status are also associated with predominantly manual occupational classes—high maternal mortality, high mortality in the first year of life, high incidence of low-birthweight babies, and high absence from work through sickness. The more limited information (from the General Household Survey) shows a pattern for morbidity qualitatively similar to that for mortality; and in industrial societies generally there is a gradient both of mortality and morbidity related to occupational status.

The national occupational classes are each made up of a considerable number of occupations, which may differ from one another in ways other than socioeconomic status. This has led to studies of people in single organizations, but with gradations in status within them. Both in the civil service and in the British Army (in peacetime), mortality is higher among lower-ranking members than among those in the upper echelons. Results from longitudinal studies are beginning to become available and in terms of mortality are in accord with the cross-sectional national findings. Studies have been carried out using various indicators of deprivation and health status in defined local government areas in Edinburgh, Glasgow, Sheffield, Bristol, Newcastle, and London. The results have consistently shown both mortality and morbidity to be increased with increase in measures of the deprivation of the area. Individual facets of deprivation that are demonstrably linked with poor health include unemployment; housing that is crowded, of poor quality, and rented rather than owned; single parenthood; lack of safe facilities for recreation (especially for children and young adults); eligibility for social benefits subject to a means test; and lack of a car. Perhaps surprisingly, in one study "the strongest association between health and deprivation variables was with lack of a car."[7]

There has been continued interest in international comparisons, although in relation to both social deprivation and health, whatever variations are found within industrial countries are indeed small in comparison with the gulf between them and the countries of the Third World, which are crushed by burdens of overpopulation, famine, civil and international strife, and all manner of disease. I question the value of international comparisons in relation to the problems that are the subject of this chapter. Countries and their inhabitants differ in so many ways as to make analysis, whether of economics or of health, extremely confused. And it is hard to go beyond the generalization, already deducible from what can be learned in one country, that where there are degrees of deprivation, there are also corresponding degrees of ill-health. Two of the countries that have the most favorable life expectancy are Japan and Sweden. Tokyo is the "healthiest" city in the world, and Sweden's health may be partly related to a higher level of deliberate social welfare provision.

An important study has just been published reporting the results of applying the newer techniques of area-based analysis of deprivation and of health to Scotland, with its population of a little more than 5 million.[8] More than 1,000 areas defined by postal code offered a wide range of populations living under different social conditions. The index of deprivation, derived from census information, was based on four variables—overcrowding at home, unemployment, car ownership, and social class as defined on OPCS criteria. Health records for the same areas gave information on mortality, hospital admissions, births in hospital, registered cancers, and absence from work resulting from temporary or long-lasting ill-health. As in other studies, mortality was higher in the more deprived areas throughout the life span. Low-birthweight babies were twice as common in the most deprived areas, thereby partially accounting for the higher perinatal and infant mortality in deprived areas. Temporary sickness was six times as common and permanent sickness three times as common in the most deprived as compared with the least deprived areas. Although the ratio relating most deprived to least deprived areas for all cancers was 1.3, that for cancer of the lung was 2.9. It is, of course, most likely that the high ratio for lung cancer reflected smoking habits. Smoking is also a risk factor for ischemic heart disease, but the ratio for that condition was only 1. 3 for all ages and 2.0 for ages 0–64, showing the diluting effect of risk factors other than smoking. This large-scale study, as much as any other, seems to put beyond reasonable doubt a strong association between socioeconomic deprivation and ill-health, and there is indeed what almost amounts to a consensus that the association is real. But consensus vanishes the moment explanations for the association are sought; and there is even greater discord relating to what, if anything, should be done about it.

Explanations

Evidence derived from a wide range of social settings and using a variety of epidemiological methods has established a convincing association between socioeconomic circumstances and health status. The number and variety of independent studies that have demonstrated this association make it unlikely that it has arisen through mere chance. If we then look for a cause of the association, there are three obvious possibilities, not necessarily exclusive of one another:

1. Socioeconomic circumstances are an important determinant of health status.
2. Health status is a determinant of socioeconomic circumstances.
3. There is a third factor that determines both socioeconomic circumstances and health status.

Let me begin with the third possibility because it is perhaps the least likely of the three and cannot be critically examined unless this third factor has been adequately defined and measured. It has indeed been suggested that "failure to cope" may be the common cause of social deprivation and poor health,[9] but this concept is not susceptible of clear definition, still less of accurate measurement. It is of course true that individuals vary considerably in their ability to adapt to situations, and that failure to do so can lead to poverty and ill-health. But it is not easy to transfer failure to cope—an essentially individual characteristic—to the behavior of groups. In addition, this hypothesis is essentially defeatist in the sense that if socioeconomic status and health are alike dependent on primary individual inadequacy, there is little that can be done about either.

The first and second of the possible explanations are of a different order in that socioeconomic circumstances and health can be observed and to an extent measured. They are also open to interventions of various kinds, although with variable degrees of success, which depend largely on the basic social or health problem but also on the competence of the intervention. Neither socioeconomic circumstances nor health status is a completely independent variable. On the one hand, social deprivation can lead to poor health, most clearly demonstrable perhaps in the case of unemployment. On the other hand, poor health can cause a drift down the social scale. At some risk of oversimplification, the question to be asked is

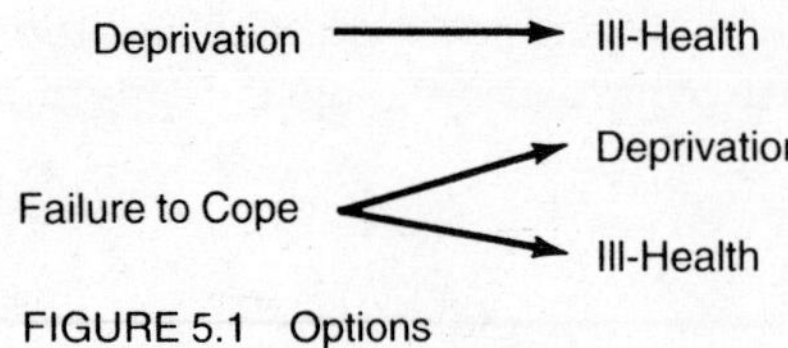

FIGURE 5.1 Options

not "Which is the independent and which the dependent variable?" but rather "Which is quantitatively the more important, the influence of deprivation as a predisposing factor to ill-health, or the influence of ill-health in inducing deprivation?" As a matter of simple observation, both these processes occur; but which is quantitatively the more important?

These issues may be made clearer if the options are set out in a diagram (see Figure 5.1). The failure to cope model is represented in the lower part of the figure. The upper part expresses what I see as the more likely model, in which the interdependence of social deprivation and ill-health is recognized but the relative length of the arrows connecting them expresses the belief that although both effects can be demonstrated, the effect of social circumstances on health is quantitatively more important than the effect of health on social circumstances.

Given the diversity of ways in which ill-health, whether physical or mental, can impair working capacity, or even lead to total loss of employment, there is little point in enumerating or describing them. Indeed, to do so would require something like a textbook of medicine. But one general point may be appropriately made in justification of our claim that the overall effect of health on social status is less important than that of social status on health: In a modern industrialized society the burden of illness falls more heavily in childhood (and especially in infancy) and in older ages than in the years of active employment. This does not mean that illness in the working years is unimportant, still less that at any age it should be neglected when effective measures are available.

The ways in which socioeconomic status can affect health are similarly diverse. But if we are correct in our beliefs that they are important and that something should be done about them, some degree of analysis is required. Evidence accumulated in recent years makes it less likely that the apparent link is due in any great degree to artifacts of measurement.[10] The possibility of health-based social mobility has to be considered—that is, healthier people move up the social scale, thereby making the upper social classes more healthy than previously, and less healthy people swell the ranks of the lower social classes. Such movement does occur, but it is insufficient to account for any major part of the association between social class and health. The same analysis of recent evidence concludes "Estimates of the size of the selection effect suggest that it accounts for only a small proportion of the overall differential between the social classes."[11] Prior illness as an explanation of the poorer health found in lower grades in the British civil service was made unlikely by the rigorous medical examination carried out on all entrants.[12]

Two types of primarily social explanations—cultural/behavioral and structural material—merit consideration. The first of these ascribes the poor health of the socially deprived to unhealthy ways of life and specifically to bad habits such as smoking (which is assuredly a cause of much illness). The second sees the stratification of society as a prime cause of ill-health associated with lower social status. These two social explanations are not mutually exclusive, and each has its dangers. Adherents of the first can come dangerously close to blaming the victim. Proponents of the second can pay insufficient regard to people's responsibility for their own health. In her recent extensive analysis of these matters, Nicky Hart—who was a research assistant to the original team and like them had strongly favored the structural/material explanation—still regards the weight of the historical, geographical, and epidemiological evidence as favoring the structural/material explanation but also concedes considerable importance to cultural factors such as education, literacy, and personal and political freedom.[13] To give a specific example, the favorable health experience of the Japanese may owe something to their high social stability, reflected in low rates of divorce and illegitimacy. She raises the intriguing question, whether "traditional kinship norms" could be re-introduced in Britain and North America, "in the face of market forces and rampant individualism."

Perhaps not; and certainly not overnight. So our meliorative attempts must be on a scale humbler than a complete recasting of society as we know it. This calls for analysis of specific mechanisms that may link deprivation (assumed to be a given in both capitalist and communist societies) and consequent ill-health. The poor are disadvantaged in health at every stage of life—even before they are born! But the links between poverty and ill-health are different at various life stages. In the womb and in infancy, the health of the offspring is largely dependent on the health of the mother and on the quality of the care she is capable of giving. Children are vulnerable largely to infections and to accidents in the home and at play—overcrowding, poor-quality housing, and lack of safety are adverse tangible factors, but the care given by parents, including adequate stimulation, is also important. (Nutrition is also especially important in childhood for growth and resistance against infection. In Britain or the United States, there is not likely to be anything approaching undernutrition, but the poor are subject to malnutrition given that protective foods are more expensive than sugars and starches.) In adult working life, deaths from all causes, although infrequent overall, are commoner in manual workers, many of whom are often engaged in dangerous or dusty occupations; and some of their increased mortality can at least be traced back to illnesses in childhood. The health disadvantage of the poor persists into old age. As we put it in our report, "The bodies of men seem to exhibit the effects of wear and tear sooner than those of women, and those of manual workers sooner than those of non-manual, and the manifestations of degeneration in disease become more frequent. What has to be remembered is that these outcomes are the end product of inequalities in the use made of, and the demands made upon, the human body earlier in the lifetime and the kind of environment in which human beings have been placed."[14]

What Can Be Done?

Once again, I wish to begin by disposing of the easiest, but also the least acceptable, response to the problem, which in this case is to do nothing. Inaction is not completely untenable, either intellectually or morally; if it were, responsible people would not be found to support it. Arguments made in support of inaction can range from a belief that low socioeconomic status reflects inbuilt individual inadequacy to a notion that social stratification is part of the divine ordering of things.

There are, however, arguments that are less insulting to the victims or to providence. In countries such as the United States and Britain that run their democracies on adversarial lines, politicians in office are conscious of the economic cost a radical solution of social inequalities might bring—in the Foreword supplied to our report by the secretary of state for social services, he claims that "a major and wide-ranging program of public expenditure capable of altering the pattern" would be "quite unrealistic in present or any foreseeable economic circumstances."[15] As a detached observer, I personally regret the extent to which the issues of poverty and health have become politically polarized in Britain, so that in one party genuine concern about ill-health associated with deprivation tends to be muted, while in other political parties it may be overemphasized.

It is also argued by those uninterested in the condition of the socially disadvantaged that the main effort should be directed to improving the circumstances of the whole nation, the consequent benefits then filtering down to the poorest in due course. It is true that the health of all social classes in Britain has improved very greatly over the past 50 years as general prosperity has increased; and it is also true that the numbers of people in unskilled manual occupations have decreased from 17.8 percent of the population in 1931 to 6 percent in 1981. Nevertheless, the magnitude of persisting inequality and indeed its probable increase do not suggest that filtering down will suffice to correct the problem;[16] and even if the numbers of the most disadvantaged are less, this does not console the remaining individual for his poor status and health, which may be further aggravated by unemployment, to which he is more liable than those in skilled occupations.

I do not believe that socially determined health inequality on the scale we have it is tolerable in a society that is comparatively affluent and that professes social concern. Nevertheless, I am unable to regard this particular health problem as of such unique importance as to displace all other health initiatives, such for example as medical research or medical aid to the developing countries. Fortunately, there is a wide enough space between indifference and obsession to leave room for sensible and affordable measures of health-related social engineering. I believe that much, if not all, of what we recommended would fall into that category. Many of the recommendations we made would not be costly, and some were applicable to the type of social and health services then enjoyed in Britain. Rather than detailing them here, I wish instead to outline a general strategy, the details of which can be divided into two main categories—socioeconomic measures and medical measures.

Socioeconomic Measures

Modern industrial societies have evolved through, and continue to require, high levels of specialization; and those skills that are both rare and in high demand are likely to attract proportionate (or should it be disproportionate?) economic rewards. This is one basis of the class system as we know it, another being the persistence of hereditary privilege that in Britain is only less refractory to change than the caste system in India. A classless society is discussed but is not likely to be experienced.

We believed that poverty brought a constellation of disadvantages, only some of which could be alleviated by secondary measures such as means-tested social benefits of various kinds. The long-term ideal must be the disappearance of extreme degrees of poverty, which would call for either a radical reconstruction of society toward greater equality or else welfare expenditure on a scale beyond the means of even the wealthiest countries. But within the limits of what can be afforded, it seems desirable to direct social benefits specifically toward those who stand most in need. Identifying those most in need has its problems, although these are not so insuperable as they may appear to those who see fraud in every claim for help.

One approach to which we gave the highest priority was to give special help to children in the most disadvantaged families—not for sentimental reasons, but on the evidence that health in childhood is a determinant of health in later life and on the hard practical consideration that a health benefit gained in childhood can be enjoyed for the rest of what may be a long lifespan. Detailed social measures that can improve child health at containable cost are safety measures at home and at play, health education in schools, health education for parents regarding accident prevention and nutrition, and provision of milk and school meals.

The direct relief of poverty certainly causes more problems of possible misappropriation than does help given directly to children. Those who administer social services and financial benefits have a hard task in identifying a family's responsible member, to whom benefits should be paid. Fiscal measures should be used to discourage expenditure of scarce resources on commodities that are themselves damaging to health—it is a sad fact that education on the dangers of smoking is less effective than an increase in the tax on tobacco products.

I have spoken of these social measures with diffidence, having no expertise in social administration; but if we are right in considering deprivation as a major cause of ill-health, then the importance of social measures must be stressed. It has indeed been claimed that this century's improvements in health have been predominantly the result of social and economic factors, with medical advances playing only a minor role.[17] This is a troubling notion for any doctor who has seen and welcomed each advance as it came along and noted the virtual disappearance in developed countries of diseases such as tuberculosis and smallpox. This idea also happens not to be entirely true. If diseases for which treatment is available (amenable diseases) are separated off from diseases for which no treatment is yet available (nonamenable diseases) the mortality from the first group has declined much more rapidly than that from the second. (Of course, there are still many more deaths from nonamenable diseases than from amenable diseases, which is not entirely surprising—medicine still has a long way to go, and in any case immortality is not a terrestrial benefit.) But over the period 1951 to 1980, this was an experience shared in Britain, Sweden, France, Italy, Japan, and the United States.[18] And it suggests that medical measures, although less important quantitatively than social measures in their potential for lessening the adverse effect of deprivation on health, are still worth considering.

Medical Measures

Although it is convenient for descriptive purposes to distinguish between socioeconomic and medical measures, they overlap to some extent, and they both consume financial and human resources. Similarly, it is convenient to separate public health or community/population medical measures from clinical measures. Since our problem was essentially related to defined populations, most of our medical recommendations related to public health, rather than to individual clinical, medicine. But there is no absolute separation of the two spheres because effective public health diminishes the incidence and consequent burden of clinical disease and effective cure of acute illness is an important way of preventing chronic illness and disability, which impose great burdens on public health resources.

The particular focus on children in our social recommendations continues in our medical ones. Surveillance of children at school should include regular assessment and recording of hearing, vision, height, and weight. Accidents involving children should be registered and analyzed to improve the information base for an educational program of accident prevention. Surveys should be made not just of what food is provided for children in school and at home, but also of what food is actually consumed. The results can then be assessed in terms of nutritional value, and if necessary, a corrective educational program can be mounted. At a still earlier stage of life, the existing gap between surveillance of infants and of schoolchildren should be closed by surveillance of preschool children. (This is one area in which progress has belatedly been made by the recent encouragement and inducement of general practitioners to complete the immunization of children at appropriate stages.) Earlier still, antenatal clinics contribute to the health of the fetus as well as to that of the mother. (In France, payment of maternity benefit is made conditional on regular attendance at antenatal clinics; but we preferred, perhaps less effectively, to retain faith in persuasion.)

We also laid stress on improved recognition of disability or handicap. This is relevant to our problem as something that can depress individuals in the social scale and that consequently has a high prevalence in socially deprived groups. We recommended more systematic registration of disabilities, with a view to rationalizing the provision of appropriate services.

Perhaps our most general recommendation, and also our most controversial one even within the group, was for a greatly expanded program of health education and of preventive measures, such as general screening for disease and active discouragement of cigarette smoking, including fiscal measures. Although we agreed on general principles, we disagreed on details and on where the needed money was to come from.

In theory at least, there is in Britain no problem of availability of medical and nursing care for any group—every citizen is entitled to be registered with a general practitioner (generalist or family doctor), who can also call on nursing and social services. Theory is not always reflected in reality, however, and there are specific problems of homelessness and inner-city disorganization. But the great majority of the people, including unskilled manual workers, do have a family doctor, and there is information on how this service is being used. The more deprived groups use the treatment services more intensively than less deprived groups do, largely because of their greater need. But they also partly fail to take up preventive services, whether these are provided by their family doctor or by community or hospital clinics. This is at least partly due to problems with transportation and loss of wages. We recommended a strengthening of community and general practitioner services to improve both access and quality. We also made a number of recommendations for research, many of which—in some contrast to our recommendations for expenditure, which we considered to be directly beneficial—have been taken up, some of them even with the support of government agencies.

Summary

There is evidence of an association between socioeconomic deprivation and ill-health. It seems clear that ill-health can lead to descent in the social scale and that socioeconomic deprivation, however caused, can have serious adverse effects on health. The second of these processes appears to be quantitatively the more important. If that is so, the problem of socially determined ill-health calls primarily for social or welfare measures; but medical measures can also make an important contribution.

Notes

1. K. Popper, *The Open Society and Its Enemies* (London: Routledge and Kegan Paul, 1945).

2. P. Townsend and N. Davidson, *Inequalities in Health: The Black Report* (London: Penguin Books, 1982).

3. M. Whitehead, *The Health Divide: Inequalities in Health in the* 1980s (London: Health Education Council, 1987); and Townsend and Davidson, *Inequalities in Health.*

4. R. G. Wilkinson, ed., *Class and Health* (London: Tavistock, 1986).

5. L. Fallowfield, *Quality of Life: The Missing Dimension in Health Care* (London: Souvenir Press, 1990).

6. Townsend and Davidson, *Inequalities in Health.*

7. Whitehead, *The Health Divide.*

8. V. Carstairs and R. Morris, *Deprivation and Health* (Aberdeen, Scotland: Aberdeen University Press, 1991).

9. D. L. Crombie, *Social Class and Health Status: Inequality or Difference,* Occasional Paper 25 (London: Royal College of General Practitioners, 1984).

10. Whitehead, *The Health Divide.*

11. Whitehead, *The Health Divide.*

12. M. G. Marmot, M. J. Shipley, and G. Rose, "Inequalities in Death Specific Explanations of a General Pattern?" *Lancet,* i(1984):1003–06.

13. N. Hart, "The Social and Economic Environment and Human Health," in W. W. Holland, R. Detels, and G. Knox, eds., *Oxford Textbook of Public Health,* 2nd ed. (Oxford: Oxford University Press, 1991).

14. Townsend and Davidson, *Inequalities in Health*.
15. Townsend and Davidson, *Inequalities in Health*.
16. Whitehead, *The Health Divide*.
17. T. McKeown, *The Role of Medicine: Dream, Mirage or Nemesis* (Oxford: Blackwell, 1979).
18. R. H. Charlton and R. Velez, "Some International Comparisons of Mortality Amenable to Medical Intervention," *British Medical Journal* i(1986):195–301.

6

Medical Care and the Poor: Focus on Hypertension and Diabetes

Nicole Lurie

Rather than focus on generic issues pertinent to providing medical care for the poor, this chapter relates issues in the health care delivery system to two chronic conditions prevalent among the poor: hypertension and diabetes. Before doing so, I wish to delineate several issues. First, we must distinguish clinical issues in caring for hypertensives and diabetics from issues regarding the system in which their care is delivered. Second, we must recognize that "the poor" are a heterogeneous group and define them further. Finally, we must bear in mind that the spectrum of disease for both hypertension and diabetes is quite broad. Although clinicians treat elevated blood pressure and glucose to avoid immediate effects of loss of control, most therapy is aimed at preventing longer term sequelae. I consider that these complications are part of the disease process itself.

Clinical Care Versus Delivery of Care

There is no doubt that there have been significant advances in the clinical care of hypertensives and diabetics in the past decade. First, there is an increased awareness of the severity of hypertension among certain subpopulations, notably blacks, and an appreciation of their increased risk for developing end organ disease, particularly renal failure.[1] Second, there has been an increased awareness of the need to treat systolic hypertension.[2] Finally, there have been major changes in drug therapy for hypertension. Two new classes of medications, angiotension converting enzyme inhibitors and calcium channel blockers, are now widely used. Even though they represent advances in regard to side effect profile and cardioprotection, they have also dramatically increased the cost of treating hypertension. For example, ten years ago initial treatment for hypertension began with a diuretic at a cost of less than $1 per month (1991 prices). Today, initial treatment with a long-acting calcium-channel blocker commonly costs about $30 per month.[3] This increased cost becomes an issue as we discuss access to medications.

There have been similar advances in diabetes care. There has been increased appreciation of the role of non-insulin-dependent diabetes and a recognition that certain subpopulations, particularly black women, are at increased risk of developing diabetes and its complications.[4] Again, major changes in drug therapy have occurred, and they have increased the cost of care. While they may confer a therapeutic advantage for some patients, they probably do not promote better glucose control for the diabetic population overall.

Who Are the Poor?

Rather than defining "the poor," I prefer to think of populations that are at a relative disadvantage in accessing the health care system. These include the very poor, who in many states are eligible for Medicaid or General Assistance (although eligibility varies by state), those who are poor and uninsured, and those who are poor, employed, and underinsured. We can define individuals who are underinsured as those with a chronic health condition, in this case hypertension or diabetes; those who do not have basic inpatient and outpatient coverage; or, to use Farley's definition, those who spend more than 10 percent of their income on health care.[5] These latter individuals are often low-income workers, the self-employed, part-time workers at low-wage jobs, or rural residents. In Minnesota, this figure is 25–33 percent of individuals who purchase insurance on their own (i.e., not through a group or an employer).[6]

Race is frequently used as a surrogate measure of poverty status because nonwhite populations often have lower income than whites. This creates some confusion with regard to hypertension and diabetes because independent of socioeconomic characteristics, these conditions are more prevalent and severe in black populations and because the physiologic and pharmacologic responses to therapy are different in blacks and whites. Thus, when we speak of worse outcomes among blacks, we can attribute only part of the variance to poverty and its associated problems with access to care. Nevertheless, examining racial differences can tell us something about access to care.

Access to Care

Access to care is defined by Andersen et al. as "those dimensions which describe potential and actual entry of a given population to the health care delivery system."[7] They further distinguish among predisposing, need, and enabling aspects of access to care. Predisposing factors are those qualities indigenous to the individual that affect his or her propensity to approach or use the health care system, such as age, ethnicity, cultural beliefs, or gender. Need factors are those factors such as health status or level of distress of the individual. Enabling factors are those that facilitate entry into the health care system and include insurance status, income, and geographic distance to the provider.

The poor experience barriers to access on all three levels. First, as a group they are less well educated than their more affluent counterparts, and this may serve to inhibit them from dealing with the organizational barriers necessary to access the health care system or to use it effectively. Second, they are likely to be discriminated against not only because they are more likely to be ethnic minorities, but also because they are more likely to be members of other "stigmatized" groups, such as those with chemical dependency, mental illness, or HIV-related problems. Third, poor individuals report worse perceived health status and more chronic illness than the nonpoor do.[8] Thus, their needs are higher. As Andersen et al. point out when they define equity of access to care as "services that are distributed on the basis of people's need for them," the poor often have higher needs than the nonpoor. Thus, merely finding evidence of similar use of services between poor and nonpoor groups does not imply equitable access. Fourth, the poor are less likely to have adequate insurance or a regular source of care.

Both financial and nonfinancial barriers can manifest differently in varying geographic areas. For example, among those uninsured in Minnesota who reported being refused care, the overwhelming majority lived in urban areas.[9] Furthermore, uninsured rural individuals were less likely than urban dwellers to report delays in care and were more likely to have a regular source of care. The social nature of the community in which low-income individuals live may have some effect on their access to care. Poor individuals living in rural areas may have difficulty locating a geographically convenient provider or hospital, but if there is a provider in a small community, he or she may be less likely to discourage an individual without financial resources from seeking care elsewhere. In urban areas, care is provided by individuals working in large organizations, rather than by individual providers. There are often places of "last resort" to which providers may refer patients, particularly those who are unfamiliar and do not have the resources to pay. Likewise, patients are more anonymous and not known by providers in the community.

Although a discussion of all access barriers is beyond the scope of this chapter, I focus on those that are amenable to remedy by alterations in health policy or by other interventions. For this reason, I stress financial access to care as it can be improved once there is a national will to enact one of multiple proposals for "universal access." I do not discuss those that might be altered by changes in social and economic policy designed to reduce or eliminate poverty.

Evidence of Threatened Access to Care

In addition to the foregoing reasons that the poor may have less access to care, several studies point to reduced access to care for low-income diabetics and hypertensives. First, a recent report from the Centers for Disease Control indicates that 1988 mortality rates for blacks, which had been falling, are now increasing.[10] Compared with 1987, age-adjusted death rates fell for whites but increased for blacks, from 778.6 to 788.8 per 100,000 population. Major causes of death included heart disease and stroke, where the ratio of black to white death rates were 1.4 and 1.9, respectively. Not all of the excess stroke mortality in blacks can be attributed to differences in prevalence of hypertension among blacks and whites.[11] There is increasing concern that deteriorating access to care is an important factor in explaining these differences.

In a study of hypertensives in Georgia, Shulman et al. highlighted the problem of financial access to medications for blacks and its link to poor blood pressure control.[12] In their study, a larger proportion of uncontrolled moderate to severe hypertensives reported cost of medicines as a problem "all or most of the time" than those with mild or controlled hypertension. These problems were most pronounced among black women, of whom 42 percent with uncontrolled blood pressure reported financial problems; 54 percent of those treated with medicine reported times when they were unable to afford a prescription refill for antihypertensive medicines.

Lack of access to primary care remains a problem for low-income individuals, as new kinds of evidence are demonstrating. For example, building on the work of Rutstein in developing sentinel health events, Billings et al. recently specified a set of conditions for which a hospitalization was likely to imply failure of ambulatory care and analyzed data on hospitalization rates for these ambulatory care sensitive (ACS) diagnoses.[13] One of these indicators was complications of diabetes such as cellulitis, diabetic ketoacidosis, and coma. Grouping New York City into zip codes, these investigators found a higher proportion of admissions for ACS conditions in zip codes with a higher percentage of people living in poverty (and also with a higher proportion of problems with alcohol and drug abuse). They suggest that the poor continue to have problems with access to ambulatory care and are hospitalized only when their problems become dangerous (e.g., DKA) or when complications of their chronic diseases develop. Similar findings have now been reported by Epstein et al., who, using Maryland data, report higher rates of hospitalization among the uninsured for conditions that could represent failures of access to ambulatory care.[14] Fisher et al. in New Hampshire report that low-income areas of New Hampshire also have higher than expected admission rates for a similar set of conditions.[15]

Even though these data again suggest that access barriers result in adverse outcomes in the form of increased hospitalization, they leave some unanswered questions. For example, are doctors more likely to admit a low-income patient than a middle-class patient to the hospital because of concerns about access or compliance or fears that the problem will progress without care? We also know that the poor are sicker and that the prevalence of ACS diseases may simply be higher in low-income areas. More detailed investigations of this phenomenon are now under way.

Financial access to care, either through insurance or some other mechanism, is usually a prerequisite to treatment. Here I review the most prevalent mechanisms by which financial access to care may be threatened: loss of insurance or source of care, cost sharing, capitation, and discrimination in insurance. These are summarized in Table 6.1. Most of the evidence regarding these mechanisms involves basic care of hypertension and diabetes, rather than care of their complications.

It should be stressed that care of chronic conditions is unlike acute care, in which access to and use of a hospital or a procedure may be sufficient for a satisfactory outcome. Treatment of chronic conditions extends beyond the providers' office. The setting is less controlled, and the outcome more often depends upon a partnership between the provider and the patient, which for hypertension and diabetes involves the use of chronic medications. Thus, financial access to medications (and other factors that contribute to compliance with recommended treatment) may be as important as access to the provider and to tests.

Loss of Insurance or Source of Care

Several studies have examined the effects of losing insurance or financial access to a regular care source. In 1982, California terminated its Medi-Cal Program for medically indigent adults.[16] Affected individuals, who were largely the working poor, no longer received financial coverage for medical care and were forced to rely on an already overtaxed county system. A study of 186 patients previously cared for in a teaching hospital clinic demonstrated deterioration in blood pressure control for a group of hypertensives who were affected by this change, as evidenced by a ten-millimeter deterioration in diastolic blood pressure. Similar findings were not seen in a comparison group of patients. This degree of change in-

TABLE 6.1
Financial Barriers to Accessing Care for Hypertension and Diabetes: Selected Studies

Barrier/Facilitor	*Study*	*Findings*
Financial access to medications	Shulman et al.	Inability to pay for medications associated with worsened blood pressure control; problems most severe in black women
Poverty (otherwise not specified	Soumerai et al.	Three-drug limit for Medicaid-covered pharmaceuticals associated with 54 percent increase in nursing home admissions; less insulin use
Loss of insurance and/or source of care	Billings et al.	Higher rate of admissions for diabetes and related complications in New York City census tracts with a higher proportion
	Lurie et al.	Poorer control of hypertension and diabetes among patients whose Medicaid was terminated
	Fihn and Wicher	Poorer blood pressure control among Veterans terminated from VA care
	Bindman et al.	Reduced access to provider and medications and worsened health status among patients whose rural county hospital closed
	Sacerdote et al.	Worsened glucose control after a community clinic diabetes program cut
Cost sharing	Brook et al.	Better blood pressure and vision for low-income RAND HIE enrollees receiving free care
Capitation	Keeler et al.	Low-income individuals on free-care plan had 3.3mm Hg lower diastolic blood pressure than those on cost sharing
	Udvarheli et al.	No difference in blood pressure control for hypertension in HMO FFS care
	Coffey et al.	No difference in process of care for diabetes or hypertensives assigned to HMOs of FFS Medicaid
	Lurie et al.	No difference in blood pressure or diabetes control for Medicaid patients in HMO vs. FFS care

creased the relative risk of dying by 40 percent in the terminated group. One of the five deaths in the study cohort was directly attributable to the patient's inability to afford her antihypertensive medicines, resulting in a fatal stroke. Many patients reported inability to pay for medications after their Medi-Cal was discontinued. In that same study, a significant deterioration in diabetes control was also evident six months after termination from Medi-Cal, but the difference was no longer statistically significant after a year.[17] Nevertheless, intervention by the investigators on behalf of some acutely ill diabetic patients probably obscured the true level of deterioration.

Fihn and Wicher examined the outcomes of care for hypertensives who could no longer receive care through the Veterans Administration because of funding cutbacks. Their findings were nearly identical.[18] The ten-millimeter increase in diastolic blood pressure was accompanied by patient reports of inability to pay for visits and problems accessing medications.

The network of hospitals that cares for a disproportionate share of the poor has been threatened by closure of some public hospitals. Decreased access to care was documented in one such closure when Bindman et al. followed a cohort of individuals whose public hospital closed and compared them to people in counties whose hospitals remained open.[19] While the investigators did not look specifically at individuals with hypertension or diabetes, they did document that the proportion of individuals missing medication doses increased by 10 percent. Furthermore, individuals reporting access problems also reported declines on four of six dimensions of the Medical Outcome Study Short Form.[20] They also found that even individuals on Medicaid experienced significant difficulty obtaining care after the closure. Finally, a study by Sacerdote associated funding cutbacks for diabetes services in a community clinic with a significant increase in glycosolated hemoglobin, or worsened blood sugar control, among patients who attended that clinic.[21]

Cost Sharing

Financial access to care means more than simply having insurance. It means having insurance that covers conditions for which the individual needs care and that the provider will accept as payment. Access also means that the individual must not face a financial risk or commitment so burdensome that it serves as an inappropriate barrier to access each time care is sought. Even though cost sharing can contribute positively to controlling health care costs, it also has the potential to create a financial burden.

The most common forms of cost sharing are deductibles associated with insurance policies, which must be expended before insurance pays for care, and cost-sharing arrangements in which an individual pays some amount in addition to the contribution of insurance each time care is sought. This may take the form of a co-payment (for example, the individual pays $10 out of pocket for each office visit) or co-insurance (for example, the individual pays 20 percent of billed charges, and the insurance policy pays the rest). Thus, it should be obvious that even the insured can face financial barriers to access. The poorer the individual is, the more likely it is that deductibles and cost sharing will create obstacles to obtaining needed services.

The most comprehensive study of cost sharing was the RAND Health Insurance Experiment (HIE), a randomized trial of free care versus cost sharing conducted in six U.S. cities.[22] Although the study found significantly less utilization of inpatient and outpatient services among groups exposed to cost sharing, the investigators found few differences in health outcomes between groups receiving free care and those with cost sharing. There were, however, differential effects on poor and nonpoor individuals.[23] Even though the HIE attempted to oversample low-income populations, it was not a study of the poor, and there were few low-income enrollees. Relatively few individuals were treated with antihypertensive medications. Despite this, for those in the lowest third of the income distribution, free care was accompanied by an improvement in blood pressure control compared to groups that paid a portion of their medical expenses through cost sharing. Keeler et al. detailed the mechanisms through which better control of hypertension was achieved for low income individuals.[24] Free care was accompanied by more outpatient visits, leading to increased frequency of diagnosing hypertension. This case finding was accompanied by treatment and subsequently by improved blood pressure control. At each step, low-income enrollees receiving free care did better than those on cost-sharing plans. It appears, however, that most of the effect of free care was related to access to provider services.

In addition to the cost sharing discussed in the RAND HIE, many people with insurance, particularly through the individual market, experience other forms of cost sharing. In an effort to keep premium costs down, they purchase policies with large deductibles and often do not have coverage or medications.[25] This occurs more freqeuntly among low-income individuals, for whom routine care for chronic conditions such as hypertension and diabetes may be financially more difficult to obtain and for whom medication compliance is especially important. It should also be noted that coverage for preexisting conditions such as diabetes and hypertension is often excluded from such policies and that there are often waiting periods before care for a preexisting condition can be covered.

Capitation

Both public and private insurers have turned to capitation and managed care as ways to control health care costs. Theoretically, individuals with chronic illnesses such as diabetes and hypertension could benefit from such arrangements in that care for these conditions may be better coordinated than in the traditional fee-for-service system. Nevertheless, capitated providers have a clear incentive to do less for any given patient. Schlesinger articulates the problems that could arise from such arrangements and argues that the poor and chronically ill may suffer in such a system. Two recent studies describe the care of hypertensives in HMOs. In the first, Udvarhelyi and colleagues examined the quality of care for individuals who chose to enroll in one of several HMOs or in fee-for-service care.[26] While the authors found slightly more preventive behaviors in the HMO group, there was no difference in blood pressure control. The individuals studied were not poor, however, and there was self-selection into HMO and fee-for-service care. Coffey et al. examined treatment of hypertensive and diabetic elderly Medicaid clients who were randomly assigned to HMO and fee-for-service care during the Medicaid demonstration project in Hennepin County, Minnesota.[27] They postulated that HMO patients might be prescribed less expensive medications than fee-for-service patients and that there would be a greater emphasis on dietary and lifestyle counseling. But they were unable to find any difference in pharmacologic therapy between the two groups. Specifically, once patients were enrolled in HMOs, their providers did not alter their therapeutic regimens to make care less expensive. Disappointing, however, was the finding that there were no differences between HMO and fee-for-service care with regard to dietary counseling or advice regarding smoking, weight loss, salt intake, or exercise for either diabetic or hypertensive patients. In a related study of the same population, Lurie et al. found no differences in glucose or blood pressure control for diabetics or hypertensives, respectively, a year after assignment to HMO or fee-for-service care.[28]

In this context it is important to note that an increasing number of states are experimenting with capitated care for their Medicaid clients.[29] Thus, the quality of care that Medicaid clients receive in HMOs is likely to receive increasing attention.

Access to Care in Medicare and Medicaid

By and large, individuals covered by Medicare are not considered to have significant problems accessing care. Nevertheless, a sizable portion of the Medicare population lives not only on a fixed, but also on a low, income. Thus, the financial barriers related to co-payments and deductibles may operate for this subgroup of Medicare beneficiaries. Furthermore, in the absence of a supplemental policy or Medicaid, Medicare does not pay for medications including antihypertensive and hypoglycemic agents, the implications of which have been previously discussed.

Even though Medicaid has historically played a major role in increasing access to care, Medicaid payment rates in many areas have fallen to the point that providers are unwilling to accept Medicaid patients.[30] Thus, although Medicaid may pay for medications, access to providers for basic care of chronic conditions is becoming more difficult in many states.

Medicaid programs in nearly all states are experiencing serious escalation in costs, and in addition to capitation, some are imposing other limits on eligibility and services. Recently, Soumerai et al. reported on the consequences of Medicaid changes in New Hampshire that resulted in a three-drug limit on Medicaid-covered drugs.[31] Institution of this cap was associated with a 30 percent drop in the number of prescriptions filed, including a 28 percent decrease in prescriptions for insulin, which were uncompensated for by increases in prescription size. These changes were temporally linked with a 54 percent increase in the rate of admission to nursing homes. When the drug cap was replaced with a $1 co-payment per prescription, use returned to near normal levels and the rate of nursing home admissions reverted to their previous levels. These findings highlight the fact that administrative or policy changes in aid programs can be accompanied by unexpected and unintended adverse effects.

Discrimination in Insurance

The past decade has seen a significant change in third party coverage for health insurance. After the period in which HMOs selected enrollees with the healthiest risk profiles, a practice known as "skimming," the insurance industry underwent a significant increase in underwriting activity. Indeed, such activity now constitutes a significant proportion of the "administrative cost" of insurance. Individuals with chronic conditions such as hypertension and diabetes may be affected in several ways. First, they may be denied insurance because of such a health history. Second, they may be offered coverage but not for the preexisting chronic conditions for which they have received care. Finally, they may be offered insurance but will have to pay a significantly higher rate for their policy than those without preexisting conditions. Indeed, in hearings of the Minnesota Health Care Access Commission, individuals with these chronic conditions or a family history of them testified about being denied insurance for these reasons. This is more likely to affect the working poor, who are often in small business labor markets that are less protected from underwriting.

Nonfinancial Barriers to Access

Much has been written about nonfinancial barriers to access to care, and these have recently been well outlined by Ginzberg and Ostow.[32] Although a discussion of all of these barriers is beyond the scope of this review, I highlight two potential barriers associated with racial differences and problems in patient-doctor communication.

Treatment of complications of disease serves to illustrate the former. As already discussed, the complications of diabetes and hypertension can include stroke, cardiovascular disease, and renal failure. Progression to these complications is more rapid and severe in blacks, but these problems also result from inadequate control of the disease process at an early stage. We have already seen that access to care is important in controlling hypertension and diabetes and that the poor are less likely to have access to such care.

Care for complications of diabetes and hypertension often involves hospitalization and high-cost, high-technology procedures such as cardiac catheterization and revascularization and dialysis. Several recent studies have found that, after adjusting for severity of heart disease, blacks (and women) were less likely to undergo cardiac catheterization in the setting of a myocardial infarction, a condition for which hypertension and diabetes are risk factors.[33] Kasiske et al. and Kjellstrand and Logan also found that although a higher proportion of blacks than whites were on dialysis because of a higher prevalence of end-stage renal disease, there was evidence of decreased access to dialysis and renal transplantation.[34] In none of these studies is the issue clearly an economic one. Once age, sex, severity of disease, and insurance status are controlled for, the differential findings for race persist. It is noteworthy that this is not only the case for complications of hypertension and diabetes. Durbin et al. found that for leukemics older than age 21, individuals with private insurance and those who are white are more likely to receive bone marrow transplantation.[35]

There are several possible explanations for these findings. First, blacks (and women) may have different preferences for treatment than whites (or men)—that is, equivalent patients confronted with the same clinical situation choose different forms of therapy, and this varies with ethnicity or gender. Another is that doctors distinguish between patients according to gender and ethnicity and are less aggressive about offering high-tech care to the latter groups or view their problems with different levels of seriousness. Thus, one particular area that deserves future attention is understanding how preferences for given treatments (and for health care in general) differ for population subgroups.

In addition to the aforementioned therapies, new treatments for complications of diabetes and hypertension are rapidly becoming available. For example, heart transplants have been performed on individuals with hypertensive cardiomyopathy, and pancreas and pancreatic islet transplants will probably soon emerge as treatments for diabetes. I mention these because they are also expensive therapies, and because low-income uninsured and some publicly insured individuals with diabetes may not gain access to these newer therapies, just as they appear to have unequal access to other high-cost technologies now. Furthermore, states that apply other rationing techniques (e.g., Oregon Health Decisions) to low-income or Medicaid populations may differentially deprive the poor of access to such therapies.[36]

Interventions to Increase Access to Care

Will improving financial access to care improve blood pressure or diabetes control or prevent complications? How much financial help is enough? We are currently evaluating several pilot health insurance programs that have begun to enroll low-income uninsured populations in the state of Minnesota. One of these programs provides discounted fee-for-service care to low-income individuals up to 200 percent of the federal poverty limit on a sliding scale. We compared blood pressures in 86 hypertensives before and after their enrollment in this program.[37] Overall, there were no changes in blood pressure control in the group from enrollment to one year later. Even though more hypertensives reported having at least one visit after enrollment, there were also no changes in the average number of visits or in the frequency of laboratory tests appropriate to monitoring care for hypertension. Problems with medication compliance were noted with similar frequency before and after hypertensives enrolled in the program.

The most likely explanation for these results is that the discounted fee-for-service care, up to 75 percent of the billed charges, was not a sufficient discount to remove the financial access barrier for low-income individuals. In fact, in the first year, 25 percent of the individuals enrolled in this program were terminated because of failure to pay their bills. Other explanations include the persistence of nonfinancial barriers to access and the possibility that those who enrolled were a particularly concerned group of individuals who had already achieved good blood pressure control despite financial hardship. This latter explanation clearly does not apply to the 20 percent of enrollees who had poor blood pressure control at the outset.

Florida recently discontinued a free insulin distribution for diabetes. Wylie-Rosett et al. examined the consequences of discontinuing this program and found that following cessation of the free distribution, fewer patients had glucose values over 300.[38] They also noted that the overall number of units of insulin taken by individuals was significantly less. In interpreting these latter findings, we must take into account several factors. First, the difference in blood sugar control between the pre- and postperiods, while statistically different, was not clinically meaningful. Second, evidence of "no difference" should not be interpreted as "no need." Yet it is possible that the program was targeted at individuals with less need for it than others. Finally, because insulin-dependent diabetes has different acute consequences than non-insulin-dependent diabetes, most diabetics may have recognized that they had no choice but to take insulin, and so they scraped together financial resources with which to purchase it, perhaps at the expense of something else.

Another important nonfinancial access barrier is suboptimal doctor-patient communication. This may be particularly difficult for individuals with low income or educational levels. Kaplan, Greenfield, and Ware tested an intervention designed to improve patient-doctor communication and found that patients who received the intervention exerted more control during the office visit and were more effective at obtaining information from their doctors.[39] They also found an improvement in blood glucose control as manifested by lower glycosylated hemoglobin levels and enhanced self-reported quality of life at follow-up. Would a program that provided universal access to care alleviate the problems experienced by disadvantaged populations when they need care? Certainly the financial barriers would disappear—lack of ability to pay would no longer impede care seeking or taking of medicines. But nonfinancial barriers would still exist, generated by the provider and the patient as well as by poverty. Continued attention to their causes and solutions will be crucial.

Summary

The past decade has seen many changes in the health care delivery environment. While many have affected financial access to care, and thus, health outcomes, others are likely to affect the health of diabetics and hypertensives by changing the organizational climate in which care occurs. The poor continue to be affected by these changes. Because they begin with a higher burden of illness and have worse outcomes, they deserve special attention.

Notes

1. T. J. Thom and W. B. Kannel, "Downward Trend in Cardiovascular Mortality," *Annual Review of Medicine* 32(1981):427–434; M. Feinleib, "The Magnitude and Nature of the Decrease in Coronary Heart Disease Mortality," *American Journal of Cardiology* 54(1984):2c–6c; National High Blood Pressure Education Program Working Group on Risk and High Blood Pressure, "An Epidemiological Approach to Describing Risk Associated with Blood Pressure Levels," *Hypertension* 7(1985):641; Hypertension Detection and Follow-Up Program Cooperative Group, "Five-Year Finding of the Hypertension Detection and Follow-Up Program: 1. Reductions in Mortality of Persons with High Blood Pressure Including Mild Hypertension," *JAMA* 242(1979):2562–2571; C. Sempos, R. Cooper, M. G. Kovar, and McMillen, "Divergence of the Recent Trends in Coronary Mortality for the Four Major Race-Sex Groups in the United States," *American Journal of Public Health* 78(1988):1422–1427; G. W. Comstock, "An Epidemiologic Study of Blood Pressure Levels in a Biracial Community in the Southern United States," 65(1951):271–315; N. B. Shulman, "End-Stage Renal Disease in Hypertensive Blacks," *Journal of Clinical Hypertension* 3(1987): 85s–88s; and S. G. Rostand, G. Brown, K. A. Kirk, E. A. Rutsky, and H. P. Dustan, "Renal Insufficiency in Treated Essential Hypertension," *New England Journal of Medicine* 320(1989):684–688.

2. Shep Cooperative Research Group, "Prevention of Stroke by Antihypertensive Drug Treatment in Older Persons with Isolated Systolic Hypertension: Final Results of the Systolic Hypertension in the Elderly P, *Journal of the American Medical Association* 265(1991):3255–3264.

3. V. A. Cardinale, ed., *Red Book* (Medical Economics Company).

4. H. Rifkin, and D. Porte, Jr., eds., *Diabetes Mellitus: Theory and Practice* (Elsevier Press, 1990).

5. P. J. Farley, "Who Are the Underinsured?" *Milbank Memorial Fund Quarterly/Health and Society* 63(1985):476–503.

6. N. Lurie, M. F. Finch, and B. Dowd, "Who Are the Uninsured in Minnesota?" A Report to the Minnesota Health Care Access Commission, 1990.

7. R. M. Andersen, L. A. Aday, C. S. Lyttle et al., "Ambulatory Care and Insurance Coverage in an Era of Constraint, Center for Health Administration Studies." Continuing CHAS Research Series No. 35 (Pluribus Press, 1987).

8. D. Rowland and B. Lyons, "Triple Jeopardy: Rural, Poor, and Uninsured." *Health Services Research* 23(1989):975–1004.

9. D. Hartley and N. Lurie, "Urban/Rural Differences in Access and Insurance" (unpublished ms.).

10. Mortality and Morbidity Weekly Review, *Mortality Patterns—United States, 1988.*

11. S. J. Kittner, L. R. White, K. G. Losonczy, P. A. Wolf, and J. R. Hebel, "Black-White Differences in Stroke Incidence in a National Sample: The Contribution of Hypertension and Diabetes Mellitus."

12. N. B. Shulman, B. Martinez, E. Brogan et al., "Financial Cost as an Obstacle to Hypertension Therapy," *American Journal of Public Health* 76(1986):1105.

13. D. D. Rutstein, W. Berenberg, T. C. Chalmers, C. G. Child, A. P. Fishman, and E. B. Perrin, "Measuring the Quality of Medical Care: A Clinical Method," *New England Journal of Medicine* 294(1976):582–588; and J. Billings and V. Harrelblad, "Use of Small Area Analysis to Access the Performance of the Outpatient Delivery System in New York City" (Lyme, N.H.: Codman Research Group, 1989).

14. A. M. Epstein, C. Gatsonis, and J. S. Weissman, "Is There a Link Between Insurance Status and Poor Health Outcomes? Rates of Avoidable Hospitalizations in Massachusetts and Maryland."

15. E. S. Fisher, C. Fleming, H. Sox, G. Goodman, and E. Hamilton, "Monitoring the Effectiveness of Medical Care in Meeting Public Health Needs in Northern New England: A Population-Based Approach Relying on Administrative Databases" (Paper presented at the annual meeting of the Health of the Public, September 1991).

16. N. Lurie, N. B. Ward, M. Shapiro, and R. H. Brook, "Termination from Medi-Cal: Does It Affect Health?" *New England Journal of Medicine* 311(1984):480.

17. N. Lurie, N. B. Ward, M. Shapiro, C. Gallego, R. Vaghaiwalla, and R. H. Brook, "Termination from Medi-Cal: One Year Later," *New England Journal of Medicine* 314(1986):1266–1268.

18. S. D. Fihn and J. B. Wicher, "Withdrawing Routine Outpatient Medical Services: Effect on Access and Health," *Journal of General Internal Medicine* 3(1988):356–362.

19. A. B. Bindman, D. Keane, and N. Lurie, "A Public Hospital Closes: Effects on Access to Care and Health Status," *Journal of the American Medical Association* 264(1990):2899–2904.

20. A. L. Stewart, R. D. Hays, and J. E. Ware, "The MOS Short-Form General Health Survey: Reliability and Validity in a Patient Population," *Medical Care* 26(1988):724–732.

21. S. D. Sacerdote, "Impact of Budget Cuts on Diabetic Control in Urban Adult Diabetes Clinic," *Diabetes Care* 11(1988):302–303.

22. J. P. Newhouse, W. F. Manning, C. N. Morris, L. L. Orr, N. Duan, E. B. Keeler et al., "Some Interim Results from a Controlled Trial of Cost Sharing in Health Insurance," *New England Journal of Medicine* 305(1981):1501–1507.

23. R. H. Brook, J. E. Ware, and W. H. Rogers, "Does Free Care Improve Adults' Health?: Results from a Randomized Controlled Trial," *New England Journal of Medicine* 309(1983):1426–1434; and N. Lurie, W. Manning, C. Peterson, G. Goldberg, C. Phelps, and L. Lillard, "Preventive Medicine: Do We Practice What We Preach?" *American Journal of Public Health* 77(1987):801–804.

24. E. B. Keeler, R. H. Brook, G. A. Goldberg et al., "How Free Care Reduced Hypertension in the Health Insurance Experiment," *Journal of the American Medical Association* 254(1985):1926–1931.

25. Epstein, Gatsonis, and Weissman, "Is There a Link Between Insurance Status and Poor Health Outcomes?"

26. I. S. Udvarhelyi, K. Jennison, R. S. Phillips, and A. M. Epstein, "Comparison of the Quality of Ambulatory Care for Fee-for-Service and Prepaid Patients," *Annals of Internal Medicine* 115(1991):394–400.

27. C. Coffey, N. Lurie, I. Moscovice, M. Finch. and J. Christianson, "Management of Hypertension and Diabetes in Medicaid Elderly: Does HMO Enrollment Make a Difference?" *Clinical Research* 32(1991):2.

28. N. Lurie, I. Moscovice, M. F. Finch, and J. Christianson, "HMO vs. Fee-for-Service Care: Are Outcomes Different for the Medicaid Elderly?" (unpublished ms.).

29. D. A. Freund and R. E. Hurley, "Managed Care in Medicaid: Selected Issues in Program Origins, Design, and Research." *Annual Review of Public Health* 8(1987):137–163.

30. D. E. Rogers, R. J. Blendon, and T. W. Maloney, "Who Needs Medicaid?" *New England Journal of Medicine* 309(1983):1426–1434; and K. Erdman and S. Wolfe, "Poor Health Care for Poor Americans," *Public Citizen* (1987).

31. S. B. Soumerai, J. Avorn, D. Ross-Degnan, and S. Gortmaker, "Payment Restrictions for Prescription Drugs Under Medicaid: Effects on Therapy, Cost, and Equity, *New England Journal of Medicine* 317(1987):550–556.

32. E. Ginzberg and M. Ostow, "High-Tech Medicine and Rising Health Care Costs," *Journal of the American Medical Association* 263(1990):1820–1822.

33. E. Ford, R. Cooper, A. Castaner et al., "Coronary Arteriography and Coronary Bypass Surgery Among Whites and Other Racial Groups Relative to Hospital-Based Incidence Rates for Coronary Artery Disease: Findings from NHDS," *American Journal of Public Health* 79(1991):437–440; M. B. Wenneker and A. M. Epstein, "Racial Inequalities of Procedures for Patients with Ischemic Heart Disease in Massachusetts," *Journal of the American Medical Association* 261(1989):253–257; and J. Z. Ayanian and A. M. Epstein, "Differences in the Use of Procedures Between Women and Men Hospitalized for Coronary Heart Disease," *New England Journal of Medicine* 325(1991):221–225.

34. B. L. Kasiske, J. F. Neylan II, R. R. Riggio et al., "The Effect of Race on Access and Outcome in Transplantation," 324(1991: 302–307; and C. M. Kjellstrand and G. M. Logan, "Racial, Sexual and Age Inequalities in Chronic Dialysis," *Nephron* 45(1987):257–263.

35. M. Durbin, "And Equal Transplants for All" (Paper presented at the Robert Wood Johnson Clinical Scholars meeting, Miami, Florida, 1988).

36. H. G. Welch and E. B. Larson, "Dealing with Limited Resources: Oregon Health Decision to Curtail Funding for Organ Transplantation," *New England Journal of Medicine* 319:171–173.

37. B. Sumner, K. Peterson, A. Pheley, E. Benavides, and N. Lurie, "Discounted Care for the Uninsured: Does It Hit the Target?" (unpublished ms.).

38. J. Wylie-Rosett, S. Engel, G. D'Eramo et al., "Delivery of Diabetes Care to Low-Income Patients: Assessment of a Federally Funded Pprogram."

39. S. H. Kaplan, S. Greenfield, and J. E. Ware, Jr., "Expanded Patient Participation in Medical Care: Effects on Blood Sugar and Quality of Life in Diabetes," *Journal of General Internal Medicine* 3(1988):448.

7

Socioeconomic Differentials in Arthritis and Its Treatment

Mary E. Charlson, John P. Allegrante, and Laura Robbins

The relationship between socioeconomic status and morbidity and mortality is well documented in the literature. Research conducted over several decades has consistently demonstrated that the distribution of wealth and other resources in society results in striking differentials in health status and access to medical care, with the burden of disease and illness falling disproportionately on those whose lives are characterized by low social class, poor housing, meaningless work, and other conditions of life that deprive individuals of access to economic and educational opportunity.[1] The study of socioeconomic factors has contributed to an understanding of the differential distribution of disease and illness and to prescriptions of social policy remedies to redress or mitigate the disparities of social structure that are associated with morbidity and mortality.

This chapter reviews what is known about the relationship of socioeconomic factors to arthritis and its treatment. Arthritis is a chronic disease of special interest for several reasons. First, arthritis is the most common chronic condition in the United States. The Health and Nutrition Examination Survey (HANES) demonstrated that about 33 percent of people have musculoskeletal complaints, with back and knee problems occurring most frequently.[2] The rates increase with age, are higher among women, and, perhaps most important, are considerably higher in the poor than in their wealthier counterparts. Second, arthritis and musculoskeletal conditions result in high rates of disability and, more than all other chronic con-

---

This work was supported by the National Institutes of Health (National Institute of Arthritis and Musculosketetal and Skin Diseases) Multipurpose Arthritis Center Program Grant 1 P60 AR38520-01A1.

ditions, create the most frequent need for assistance among older people. Arthritis is the main cause of disability in 12.3 percent of people with limited functioning; spinal curvature or back impairments affect 7.8 percent, impairments of lower extremities affect 6.1 percent, and intervertebral disk disorders affect another 4.4 percent.[3] Third, arthritis-related disability occurs more frequently in the poor. People with total family incomes of less than $10,000 are twice as likely as the total population to experience functional limitations in activities of daily living (ADL).[4] Fourth, arthritis-related disability is largely treatable or preventable. Although education and occupation are often studied as separate variables, here we treat them as equivalent surrogates for poverty because of the high degree of correlation among these variables. We also use symmetric polyarthritis as a surrogate for rheumatoid arthritis and oligoarthritis as a surrogate for osteoarthritis (OA). We conclude by arguing that improving the poor's access to medical care is likely to result in commensurate improvements in arthritis-related medical outcomes and in a reduction in the costs to society that are associated with impaired functioning.

The Relationship of Education, Income, and Arthritis

An increasing body of epidemiologic and sociologic evidence has demonstrated that the prevalence of arthritis and other diseases is related to education and income. In general, poor and less educated people have a higher prevalence of arthritis than people who are not poor. The percentage of people with documented musculoskeletal abnormalities is also significantly higher among people with less education and lower incomes. For example, among those earning less than $5,000 of annual income, 48 percent had a musculoskeletal abnormality, mostly osteoarthritis, in contrast to only 23 percent of those making $15,000 or more. Moreover, most common diseases, including back pain, arthritis, hypertension, and diabetes, are all more frequent among individuals who have not completed 9 years of formal education. Formal education of less than 8 years was reported by 28–37 percent of the people who had symmetric polyarthritis, as compared to 9–12 percent of the nonarthritis population.[5] In fact, for 35 out of 37 conditions examined, the highest rates were seen among those with less education. The differences, which range from threefold to sixfold, are not explained by age, sex, or smoking.[6] The same finding emerged from the Framingham study and was particularly strong for women.[7] Among patients with rheumatoid arthritis, education also correlated with disease severity, when the duration of the disease was controlled for.[8] Not only are other comorbid diseases more likely among people with less formal education; the overall outcomes are worse for patients with arthritis and other comorbid diseases.

Why do more poor people than middle- and upper-income people have arthritis? This question was explored in four national samples about which data on occupation and income were also gathered. Among full-time workers, the types of occupation and the income associated with the occupation related to the prevalence of arthritis. In addition to repetitious work, heavy physical exertion and dangerous conditions were all positively associated with arthritis,[9] which suggests that repeated minor physical trauma may produce arthritic changes over time. The two most common problems are back and knee problems. Back pain clearly occurs more frequently among those whose occupations require heavy lifting. Knee osteoarthritis is higher in laborers and service workers whose jobs involve both lifting heavy objects and repeated knee bending. Thus, the higher incidence of arthritis among the poor results from the kind of work poor people do in our society.

Poor people also have more severe disease at the outset and experience a worse clinical course than do the nonpoor. In rheumatoid arthritis patients, there are substantial differences in morbidity and mortality on the basis of educational attainment over 9 years. The differences observed are not explained by age, medications, functional status, or disease duration at the outset of symptoms.[10] These findings were also replicated in a study that examined short-term outcomes among patients with rheumatoid arthritis, systemic lupus erythematosus, and other connective-tissue diseases.[11] Socioeconomic status was measured by occupation, income, and education. The study showed that poor patients had a longer length of stay, higher total charges, but lower ancillary charges than private patients. Poorer patients, moreover, were more likely to have limitations of instrumental activities of daily living (IADL) at the outset than nonpoor private patients.

Additional evidence of the relationship between arthritis-related conditions and socioeconomic status comes from the experience of patients who have sustained hip fracture. In a study of hip-fracture patients whose first 100 days in a nursing home were charged to an HMO, patients covered by private insurance were much more likely to return to independent living than patients covered by traditional Medicare benefits. Patients in the latter group were 2. 7 times less likely than private HMO patients to return to the community.[12]

The Relationship of Arthritis to Disability

In addition to the clinical morbidity associated with arthritis, there is no question that arthritis produces disability and interferes with functional status. Arthritis, hip fracture, and osteoporosis rank high as causes of disability, behind only cardiovascular disease and visual impairment.[13]

Data from the Supplement on Aging (SOA) from the 1984 National Health Interview Survey show a similar pattern. Although disability generally increases with age and more chronic conditions, people with arthritis are 2 to 3 times more likely than those without arthritis to have difficulty walking, have 5 or more functional limitations, and have either ADL or IADL difficulties.[14] In the Framingham study, arthritis and back disorders were also found to be significantly related to disability.[15] Arthritis-related disability alone, however, is not only a problem in terms of its impact on functioning; disability due to arthritis is a major cause of nursing home placement in 15–30 percent of all residents without dementia.[16] Furthermore, disability is a predictor for increased mortality.[17]

According to the HANES data, in addition to having a higher prevalence of musculoskeletal problems, people with lower income and education had higher rates of moderate-severe activity restriction, and significantly more had a change in job status. These HANES data showed that the lowest income and lowest education groups had more than twice the rates of these disability indicators than the higher income groups. In SOA, for people who did not complete high school, the odds of having any difficulty walking, functional limitations, or ADL or IADL difficulties rose steeply among people with arthritis (either osteoarthritis or back disorders). The same trend for increasing disability with lower education attainment was also seen among people without arthritis. With back pain, the prevalence of disability was 4 times higher among those making less than $7,000 annually as compared to those making more than $25,000. Similarly, people with less than an eighth-grade education were 3 times more likely to be disabled from back pain than those with a college education.[18] In another study, disability from back pain was predicted by previous history of back pain, the patient's perception of whether she or he always felt sick, and the level of formal education.[19]

Poverty is an independent prospective predictor of the development of disability with arthritis. In a longitudinal study of aging that followed patients aged 70–74 for 2 years, the initial evaluation showed that those with more education and an annual family income of more than $25,000 had more intact function at baseline.[20] Importantly, the two-year follow-up data showed that education was a significant predictor of functional decline as well as arthritis, diabetes, stroke, visual problems, and falls. It should be noted, however, that arthritis and other medical problems did not always produce disability or functional impairment.

Poor people with arthritis are older, are less educated, and have less opportunity to change to less physically demanding jobs than others are. With symmetric polyarthritis, the earnings of women and men were 26 percent and 48 percent of those found in the nonarthritis population. Only about one-third of the gap was explained by arthritis; the major explanatory variable was age, with patients with arthritis being older. The combination of aging with little on-the-job training caused workers to curtail the number of hours they worked each year.[21] This result is consistent with reports of household work. Thus, lower formal education in patients with arthritis contributes independently to the earnings gap between people with and without arthritis, probably because the arthritic are less able to compensate for difficulty with the physical demands of a job.

Another study showed that the rates of work disability for people with involvement of one hip or knee were in the same range as patients with symmetric arthritis.[22] Specifically, women and men with only one joint involved had only 30 percent and 63 percent, respectively, of the earnings of people without arthritis. The ability to perform work was substantially compromised when even one joint was involved. For example, 20 percent of patients with only one involved joint were severely disabled, while 69 percent were able to continue working. The difference in earnings noted was only 20 percent attributable to arthritis; 40 percent was attributable to age, 17 percent to education, and 13 percent to comorbidity. The percent of those working fell in direct relation to the number of involved joints.

The Evidence from Disability Benefits

The foregoing makes clear that more poor people have arthritis. Moreover, of those people with arthritis, a larger incidence of disability is found among the poor. What explains this difference? Can we look to disability benefits for an answer?

The issue of labor force participation and the causes of work disability continue to be hotly debated by reasonable people in social policy circles. Although it has been politically popular recently to argue that disability benefits simply encourage workers to drop out of the labor force by providing them with a generous income and no incentive to continue working in the presence of illness, there does not appear to be much empirical evidence to support this argument. One study provided an elaborate evaluation of labor force participation and work disability in an effort to shed light on this controversy. The study, conducted in 1978, involved a national survey of disabled and nondisabled adults and showed that most men worked until about age 50, after which rates of labor force participation dropped precipitously. Of the 50 percent of white men who were out of the labor force, 43 percent claimed they were retired for health reasons. The study went on to point out that in the community at large, the nature of the work and the individual's functional capacity were the strongest determinants of labor force participation; the presence of other diagnoses, attitudes about work, and the replacement rate had the weakest impact. "Discretion over the activities and pace of the job, the level of psychological demand upon the individual at work and the interactions between these two variables all profoundly alter the probability of working."[23] Thus, the combination of low discretion and high occupational demands reduces the probability of working. The implication of this finding for economic and social policy in the context of a service economy in which employment is increasingly characterized by high demand and low control is considerably daunting. If we are to encourage people to work, the challenge before us is to create more jobs that have meaning and that offer workers a sense of control.

Is Arthritis Caused by Lifestyle?

One hypothesis that has gained popularity is that low formal education puts people at risk for lifestyles that may predispose them to arthritis and other diseases. Examples of such behavioral risk factors include high-cholesterol diets and the use of tobacco or alcohol. None of these, with the exception of obesity, however, is a risk factor for the development of arthritis. This is not surprising given that weight control is a problem in the poor elderly.[24] This suggests that focusing intervention on lifestyle is not likely to produce the same outcomes in the prevention of arthritis as have population-based approaches to alter individual behavioral risk factors in other diseases.

Another relatively weak hypothesis is that the poor experience greater social isolation or stressful life events than the nonpoor do. The density and quality of social networks and other ties to the community were found to predict mortality independent of self-reported health status, socioeconomic status, and lifestyle.[25] For example, social isolation and high life stress were shown to be strongly correlated with three-year mortality risk after myocardial infarction as well as to sudden cardiac death.[26] In the elderly poor, religion (perhaps a proxy for social connectedness) and happiness reduced the risk of mortality among those in poor health.[27]

Another theory posits that low education results in learned helplessness, which in turn compromises or causes damage to the immune system and therefore places the individual at greater risk of developing arthritis and of developing more severe disease faster.[28] Helplessness is a psychological construct incorporating three types of problems found in stressful situations: motivation, such as reduced efforts to manage tasks associated with coping; cognitively reduced or ineffective efforts to develop and initiate new and adaptive coping behaviors; and emotional deficits, such as anxiety and depression, with decreased self-esteem.[29] There are some data to suggest that in rheumatoid arthritis patients, psychological status, including depression, anxiety, and helplessness, is significantly related to joint counts. These data suggest that patients with higher scores on measures of helplessness and depression have higher joint counts.[30]

What is the effect on health of the stress associated with being poor? Not surprisingly, one study evaluating different aspects of stress demonstrated that financial strains were negatively associated with physical and emotional function.[31] In this study, 2 of the 6 markers of high life stress were a low-status job, usually in clerical, sales, service, or blue-collar work, and financial difficulty.

Other Explanations

Generally, then, the literature on utilization of health services suggests that higher income, current health insurance, and more education help enable patients to seek out and gain access to medical services and treatment.[32] In addition, individual beliefs and perceptions about susceptibility to and seriousness of disease, as well as previous or vicarious experience with disease, predispose or impede both preventive and illness-related behaviors.[33] Older people are less likely than younger people to ask for help and may be more inclined to postpone medical attention until pain or problems become unmanageable. In older persons of advanced age (older than 80), low self-perceived health status and more self-reported health problems were shown to predict high utilization of inpatient and outpatient care.[34] Such patient characteristics were of particular concern because patterns of high or low use of services tended to remain stable over time, unless access to care changed dramatically.[35]

Is access to health care still a problem for poor people? In general, care for the low-income population was shown to be highly sensitive to financial barriers and to available sources of care.[36] For example, insurance status and low income were shown to predict use of ambulatory visits.[37] One study demonstrated that among working adults who were uninsured, 22 percent had no regular source of care, 39 percent had not seen a physician in the last year, and 16 percent required but did not receive medications or other needed care.[38] Household income was also shown to be an independent predictor of access. Moreover, the nearly poor (between 100 and 150 percent of the poverty level) were shown to be only slightly better off than those below the poverty level. As a result, it is not surprising that lower-income patients tend to use hospital clinics and emergency rooms to gain access to care that is otherwise not available to them.

The principal policy response to the problem of access to care for the poor was the enactment of federal legislation that established the Medicaid program. But Medicaid—which from its inception was designed to serve the poor—has been a politically unpopular program, primarily because it has been viewed as a "welfare program," despite the actual realities of the population Medicaid serves.[39] It was shown that the closure of public hospitals throughout urban centers across the nation (which served 40 percent of patients receiving Medicaid and 20 percent of those without any form of insurance) resulted in a significant deterioration in access to care.[40] People had difficulty finding physicians who accepted Medicaid, and many simply did not seek care. Patients reporting access problems also experienced deterioration in health status. In addition, serious illness may precipitate even greater financial burdens for the poor, regardless of whether they have insurance.[41]

In response to this lack of access, poor people with arthritis increasingly forgo any effort to seek definitive evaluation and care and to treat themselves instead. Population-based studies have found that half of patients treat themselves and do not see primary-care physicians about their symptoms. In a population-based study of free-living elderly, only 20–50 percent of patients with arthritis sought treatment from primary physicians.[42] And 46 percent of those with osteoarthritis (and 30 percent of those with rheumatoid arthritis) had not consulted a physician within a five-year period. For example, among manual workers with OA, a significant percentage of those with the disease treated themselves. Such self-treated patients may seek treatment only after hearing of someone who has improved after treatment for arthritis. This is particularly true for people with the most advanced symptoms.

In addition to the problem of access, the poor who do gain access to medical care often find that it is inferior and that they are less likely to receive high-technology treatments. One study of 10 million discharge summaries from 1,200 hospitals in 1987 showed that high-cost, high-discretion procedures were much less likely to be utilized with uninsured patients. Coronary artery bypass was 29 percent less likely, hip replacement was 50 percent less likely, and knee replacement was 74 percent less likely for uninsured patients as compared with privately insured patients. Similar findings have been reported for endoscopic evaluations.[43] Data indicate that when the rate of high-technology procedures is compared by insurance category, the rates of use are higher among patients with private insurance than among those covered by Medicaid or Medicare.[44] Similar findings have emerged from studies of lung cancer treatment where there are marked disparities according to the type of insurance.[45]

Conclusion

"Societies differentiate between those goods to which all citizens have an equal right and those whose unequal distribution is either acceptable or desirable. ... The economy is based on the belief that unequal distribution is an important motivator of maximum individual contribution from which everyone ultimately benefits."[46] A corollary construct is that equalization is mainly justifiable if the long-term cost to society lessens with greater equity in distribution.

In this context, it is not difficult to understand how poverty, educational attainment, occupation, housing, nutrition, employment, and income are all inextricably intertwined with health status. There is a plethora of evidence showing that some types of employment and choice of occupation present a risk to health, and this risk is compounded by the attendant lower income, poorer nutrition, poorer housing, poorer education, and greater stress.

In general, there is now impressive evidence showing that the provision of health services is probably of less relevance to health and quality of life than features of work and the environment. But it is also true that institutions in poorer communities are financially strapped and are less able to provide care because they have less resources. We cannot escape the fact that social policies pursued during the past decade have widened the gap between upper and lower income families and their access to health insurance. Soaring health care costs have now placed basic insurance out of the reach of 40 million Americans. More people with lower incomes not only develop arthritis but also develop more severe arthritis. This, in turn, more often leads to disability and decreased independence. The reasons for this situation are complex, but the lower paying, physically demanding jobs to which the poor are consigned play an unequivocal role in this nexus.

What is also clear is that some, but not all, of the work-related arthritis is preventable. Most, however, is treatable, and certainly much disability can be prevented or at least lessened with definitive medical intervention. For example, the principal treatment for severe hip and knee arthritis is total joint replacement. Since its introduction in the United States in the late 1960s, advancements in cementing techniques and prosthetic design have resulted in improved short-term outcomes.[47] Overwhelmingly, the orthopedic literature reports that 85–90 percent of patients with total hip replacement or total knee replacement enjoy an excellent outcome; recipients of joint replacements are pain free, have near normal ambulation, and recover full functional capacity.[48] Additional studies have suggested that joint replacement is one of the most cost-effective high-technology procedures.[49] This is especially noteworthy in light of the estimates showing that the major costs of arthritis are due to impairment or loss of function rather than direct medical expenditures.[50] The implications of this for health policy are clear: We need a policy that enables a greater number of people with arthritis-related functional impairment and disability to gain the benefit of treatment. In the absence of such a policy, our society can expect to continue paying for increasingly costly long-term care and custodial services.

Our society has been slow to grapple with the socioeconomic disparities that once again increasingly characterize the delivery of and access to medical care. As health care professionals, we need to recommit ourselves to the principles of social justice and equity. If we do not, we risk forsaking an entire generation of Americans whose social station we allow to determine their potential for a quality life. Until we have a system of health care that is accessible to all, the numbers of people with severe arthritis and related disability will continue to increase.

Notes

1. D. Williams, "Socioeconomic Differentials in Health: A Review and Redirection," *Social Psychology Quarterly* 53(1990):81–99.

2. L. Cunningham and J. Kelsey, "Epidemiology of Musculoskeletal Impairments and Associated Disability," *American Journal of Public Health* 74(1984):574–579.

3. M. P. Laplante, "Data on Disability from the National Health Interview Survey, 1983–85," An InfoUse Report (Washington D.C.: National Institute on Disability and Rehabilitation Research, 1988).

4. *Healthy People* 2000: National Health Promotion and Disease Prevention Objectives (Washington D.C.: U.S. Department of Health and Human Services, Public Health Service, 1990).

5. J. Mitchell, R. Burkhauser, and T. Pincus, "The Importance of Age, Education and Comorbidity in the Substantial Earnings Losses of Individuals with Symmetric Polyarthritis," *Arthritis and Rheumatism* 31(1988):348–57.

6. T. Pincus, L. Callahan, and R. Burkauser, "Most Chronic Diseases Are Reported More Frequently by Individuals with Fewer Than 12 Years of Formal Education in the Age 18–64 United States Population," *Journal of Chronic Disease* 40(1987): 865–874.

7. J. Pinsky, P. Leaverton, and J. Stokes, "Predictors of Good Function: The Framingham Study," *Journal of Chronic Disease* 40(1987):159S–167S.

8. L. Callahan and T. Pincus, "Formal Education as a Marker of Clinical Status in Rheumatoid Arthritis," *Arthritis and Rheumatism* 31(1988):1346–1357.

9. J. P. Leigh and J. Freis, "Occupation, Income and Education as Independent Covariates of Arthritis in Four National Probability Samples," *Arthritis and Rheumatism* 34(1991):984–995.

10. T. Pincus and L. Callahan, "Formal Education as a Marker for Increased Mortality and Morbidity in Rheumatoid Arthritis," *Journal of Chronic Disease* 38(1985):973–984.

11. A. Epstein, R. Tsern, J. Tognetti, C. Begg, R. Hartley, E. Cumella, and J. Ayanian, "The Association of Patients' Socioeconomic Characteristics with the Length of Hospital Stay and Hospital Charges Within Diagnosis-Related Groups," *New England Journal Medicine* 318(1988):1579–1585.

12. J. Fitzgerald and R. Dittus, "Institutionalized Patients' Hip Fracture: Characteristics Associated with Returning to Community Dwelling," *Journal of General Internal Medicine* 5(1990):298–303.

13. L. Verbrugge, J. Lepkowski, and Y. Imanaka, "Comorbidity and Its Impact on Disability," *Milbank Memorial Fund Quarterly* 67(1989):450–484.

14. L. Verbrugge, D. Gates, and R. Ike, "Risk Factors for Disability Among U.S. Adults with Arthritis," *Journal of Clinical Epidemiology* 44(1991):167–182.

15. J. Pinsky, L. Branch, A. Jette, S. Haynes, M. Feinleib, J. Cornoni-Huntley, and K. Bailey, "Framingham Disability Study: Relationship of Disability to Cardiovascular Risk Factors Among Persons Free of Diagnosed Cardiovascular Disease," *American Journal of Epidemiology* 122(1985): 644–656.

16. A. Guccione, R. Meenan, and J. Anderson, "Arthritis in Nursing Home Residents: A Validation of Its Prevalence and Examination of Its Impact on Institutionalization and Functional Status," *Arthritis and Rheumatism* 32(1989):1546–1553.

17. A. Grand, P. Gorsclude, H. Bouquet, J. Pous, and J. L. Albarere, "Disability Psychosocial Factors and Mortality Among the Elderly in a Rural French Population," *Journal of Clinical Epidemiology* 43(1990):773–782.

18. W. Cats-Baril and J. Frymoyer, "Demographic Factors Associated with the Prevalence of Disability in the General Population," *Spine* 16(1991):671–674.

19. R. Deyo and A. Diehl, "Psychosocial Predictors of Disability in Patients with Low Back Pain," *Journal of Rheumatology* 15(1988):1557–1564.

20. V. Mor, J. Murphy, S. Masterson Allen, C. Willey, A. Razmpour, E. Jackson, D. Green, and S. Katz, "Risk of Functional Decline Among Well Elders," *Journal of Clinical Epidemiology* 42(1989):895–904.

21. Mitchell, "The Importance of Age."

22. T. Pincus, J. Mitchell, and R. Burkhauser, "Substantial Work Disability and Earnings Losses in Individuals Less Than Age 65 with Osteoarthritis: Comparisons with Rheumatoid Arthritis," *Journal of Clinical Epidemiology* 42(1989):449–457.

23. E. Yelin, "The Myth of Malingering: Why Individuals Withdraw from Work in the Presence of Illness," *Milbank Memorial Fund Quarterly* 64(1986):622–649.

24. J. Lubben, P. Weiler, and I. Chi, "Gender and Ethnic Differences in the Health Practices of the Elderly Poor," *Journal of Clinical Epidemiology* 42(1989):725–733.

25. L. Berkman and L. Syme, "Social Networks, Host Resistance, and Mortality: A Nine-Year Follow-Up Study of Alameda County Residents," *American Journal of Epidemiology* 109(1979): 186–204; L. Berkman and L. Breslow, *Health and Ways of Living* (New York: Oxford University Press, 1983); and S. Cohen and L. Syme, eds. *Social Support and Health* (New York: Academic Press, 1985).

26. W. Ruberman, E. Weinblatt, J. Goldberg, and B. Chaudhary, "Psychosocial Influences on Mortality After Myocardial Infarction," *New England Journal of Medicine* 311(1984):552–559; and W. Ruberman, E. Weinblatt, J. Goldberg, and B. Chaudhary, "Education, Psychosocial Stress and Sudden Cardiac Death," *Journal of Chronic Disease* 36(1983): 151–160.

27. D. Zuckerman, S. Kasl, and A. Ostfeld, "Psychosocial Predictors of Mortality Among the Elderly Poor," *American Journal of Epidemiology* 119(1984):410–423.

28. P. Nicassio, K. Wallston, L. Callahan, M. Herbert, and T. Pincus, "Measurement of Helplessness in Rheumatoid Arthritis," *Journal of Rheumatology* 12(1985):462–467.

29. L. Callahan, R. Brooks, and T. Pincus, "Further Analysis of Learned Helplessness in Rheumatoid Arthritis Using a Rheumatology Attitudes Index," *Journal of Rheumatology* 15(1988): 418–426.

30. J. Parker, K. Smarr, S. Walker, K. Hagglund, S. Anderson, J. Hewett, A. Bridges, and C. W. Caldwell, "Biopsychosocial Parameters of Disease Activity in Rheumatoid Arthritis," *Arthritis Care and Research* 4(1991):73–80.

31. G. Parkerson, L. Michener, L. Wu, J. Finch, L. Muhlbaier, K. Magruder-Habib, J. Kertesz, N. Clapp-Channinig, D. Morrow, A. Chen, and E. Jokerst, "Associations Among Family Support, Family Stress and Personal Functional Health Status," *Journal of Clinical Epidemiology* 42(1989): 217–229.

32. L. A. Aday, "Economic and Noneconomic Barriers to the Use of Needed Medical Services," *Medical Care* 18(1975):447–456.

33. I. Rosenstock, "Why People Use Health Services," *Milbank Memorial Fund Quarterly* 44(1966):94–124; and M. Becker, ed., "The Health Belief Model and Personal Health Behavior," *Health Education Monographs* 2(1974):324–508.

34. R. Andersen and J. Newman, "Societal and Individual Determinants of Medical Care Utilization," *Milbank Memorial Fund Quarterly* 51(1973):95–124; and N. Roos and E. Shapiro, "The Manitoba Longitudinal Study on Aging: Preliminary Findings of Health Care Utilization by the Elderly," *Medical Care* 19(1981):644–656.

35. P. Denson, S. Shapiro, and M. Einhorn, "Concerning High and Low Utilizers of Service in a Medical Care Plan and the Persistence of Utilization Levels Over a Three-Year Period," *Milbank Memorial Fund Quarterly* 37(1959):217–250; J. Mullooly and D. Freeborn, "The Effect of Length of Membership upon the Utilization of Ambulatory Care Services," *Medical Care* 17(1979):922–936; T. Wan and L. Gray, "Differential Access to Preventive Services for Young Children in Low-income Urban Areas," *Journal of Health and Social Behavior* 19(1978):312–324; and J. Alpert, M. Heagarty, L. Robertson, J. Kosa, and R. Haggerty, "Effective Use of Comprehensive Pediatric Care," *American Journal of Diseases of Children* 116(1968):529–533.

36. R. Blendon, L. Aitken, H. Freeman et al., "Uncompensated Care by Hospitals or Public Insurance for the Poor," *New England Journal of Medicine* 314(1986):1160–1163; and D. Rogers, R. Blendon, and T. Moloney, "Who Needs Medicaid?" *New England Journal of Medicine* 307(1982):13–18.

37. R. Blendon, L. Aitken, H. Freeman, and C. Corey, "Access to Medical Care for Black and White Americans: A Matter of Continuing Concern," *Journal of the American Medical Association* 261(1989):278–281.

38. R. Hayward, M. Shapiro, H. Freeman, and C. Corey, "Inequities in Health Services Among Insured Americans: Do Working-Age Adults Have Less Access to Medical Care Than the Elderly?" *New England Journal of Medicine* 318(1988):1507–1512.

39. D. Rogers, R. Blendon, and T. Moloney, "Who Needs Medicaid?"

40. A. Bindman, D. Keane, and N. Lurie, "A Public Hospital Closes: Impact on Patients' Access to Care and Health Status," *Journal of the American Medical Association* 264(1990): 2899–2904.

41. L. A. Aday and R. Anderson, "The National Profiles of Access of Medical Care: Where Do We Stand?" *American Journal of Public Health* 74(1984):1331–1339.

42. H. Valkenburg, "Epidemiology Considerations of the Geriatric Population," *Gerontology* 34(Supplement 1)(1988):2–10.

43. J. Hadley, E. Steinberg, and J. Feder, "Comparison of Uninsured and Insured Hospital Patients: Condition on Admission, Resource Use and Outcome," *Journal of the American Medical Association* 265(1991):374–379.

44. E. Ford, R. Cooper, A. Castaner, B. Simmons, and M. Mar, "Coronary Arteriography and Coronary Bypass Survey Among White and Other Racial Groups Relative to Hospital-Based Incidence Rates for Coronary Artery Disease: Findings from NHDS," *American Journal of Public Health* 79(1989):437–440; and M. Wenneker and A. Epstein, "Procedures for Patients with Ischemic Heart Disease in Massachusetts," *Journal of the American Medical Association* 261(1989): 253–257.

45. E. R. Greenberg, C. G. Chute, T. Sukel, J. A. Baron, D. H. Freenman, J. Yates, and R. Korson, "Social and Economic Factors in the Choice of Lung Cancer Treatment," *New England Journal of Medicine* 318(1988):612–617.

46. A. Smith, "Social Factors and Disease: The Medical Perspective," *British Medical Journal* 294(1987):881–883.

47. N. Johanson and C. R. Charnley, "Low Friction Arthroplasty: Past Developments and Current Practice, *Contemporary Orthopedics* 19(1989):467–471; W. Harris, J. MCarthy, and D. O'Neill, "Femoral Component Loosening Using Contemporary Techniques of Femoral Cement Fixation," *Journal of Bone and Joint Surgery* 64A(1982):1063–1067; and C. Ranawat, B. Rawlins, and V. Harju, "Effect of Modern Cement Technique on Acetabular Fixation on Total Hip Arthroplasty: A Retrospective Study in Matched Pairs," *Orthopedic Clinics of North America* 19(1988):599–603.

48. W. Harris, "Total Joint Replacement," *New England Journal of Medicine* 297(1977):650–652; and J. Noble and R. Chilton, "Total Knee Replacement: Getting Better All the Time," *British Medical Journal* 303(1991):260–261.

49. A. William, "Economics of Coronary Artery Bypass Grafting," *British Medical Journal* 291(1985):326–329.

50. W. Felts and E. Yelin, "The Economic Impact of the Rheumatic Diseases in the United States," *Journal of Rheumatology* 16(1989):867–884.

8

Making a Difference in the Health of Children

C. Arden Miller

This chapter identifies social interventions that make a difference in the health of children. The list of successes is reassuring for its length and for the growing evidence that confirms its effectiveness and illuminates its dynamics. Available material justifies book-length summations, and several have been written.[1] The nation's record, however, is disturbing for the limited expression of these interventions in consistently available community programs and in enabling public policies.

Social interventions are notoriously difficult to evaluate according to conventional rules of research empiricism. A decade ago, reductions in federal financing for many social programs were defended on the basis that evidence for their effectiveness was lacking. In the intervening years supportive evaluations began to trickle in and soon became a flood. For example, one excellent report in 1985 summarized the impact of Head Start on children, families, and communities; the review embraced 1,600 documents and 210 research publications.[2] Klerman in 1991 reviewed evidence for programs that improve the health of poor children. Her excellent review cites nearly 400 publications.[3]

The vigor of these assessments is reassuring, but note can be made that in many parts of the world impressive records of child health emerged from supportive policies grounded in consensus for social justice rather than in the findings of health care research. Both approaches are necessary; neither alone is sufficient for effective social policy. My theme suggests that effective U.S. policy for children lacks more the influence of supportive social values than of data from evaluative research. Striving for equitable participation in programs for financing and providing medical care is an important undertaking that many policymakers are addressing. These efforts will be enhanced by consideration of social interventions with impressive records of achievement on behalf of children's health, especially among the most vulnerable population groups.

Cost-Effective Interventions

A 1990 report from the Select Committee on Children, Youth, and Families summarized evidence in support of public programs that were cost-effective in promoting the health, development, nutrition, and well-being of the nation's children and their families.[4] Linking cost with effectiveness is an accurate indicator of values that importantly influence current policy. A 1985 list of eight cost-effective public programs was expanded in 1990 to twelve. The list includes the following programs:[5]

- *Special Supplemental Food Program for Women, Infants, and Children (WIC).* Participation of pregnant women, new mothers, and infants in WIC improves infants' birthweight and head circumference (an important indicator of brain development) and reduces first-year hospitalization rates. WIC includes several components—food supplementation, education, and participation in health care. The effectiveness of each component cannot be separately measured.
- *Prenatal Care.* The effectiveness of prenatal care has been difficult to document because it is rendered most abundantly to populations at lowest social and demographic risk. Routine prenatal care is a weak determinant of favorable pregnancy outcome; effectiveness strengthens for comprehensive care that includes counseling, nutrition supplementation, home visitations, and other nonmedical social supports.
- *Medicaid.* Medicaid financing has increased the participation of poor children in medical care but, given their adverse health status, not to levels comparable to nonpoor children. The Medicaid component that is most promising for poor children is Early Periodic Screening, Diagnosis, and Treatment (EPSDT). It extends benefits beyond financing to approach a service entitlement, but a small proportion of eligible children (about 20 percent) are actually served.
- *Childhood Immunization.* The health effectiveness and cost-effectiveness of childhood immunizations are well established. Basic immunizations should be completed by age 2. Reliable and timely data on immunization rates for U.S. 2-year-olds are not available, but the rates are known to be substantially beneath those for other industrialized nations (by almost 35 percent) and beneath rates for much of the developing world. Immunization rates are indicators of protection against some infectious diseases (e.g., measles) and are also considered as proxy indicators for participation in well-child care.

- *Preschool Education.* Preschool education can assure linkage with programs of developmental assessment and routine preventive medical and dental care. About 40 percent of U.S. 4-year-olds participate in preschools at on average enrollee cost of $3,000 (Head Start excepted). In contrast, nearly all 4-year-olds in many Western European countries are enrolled in preschools at an enrollee cost as low as the price of the child's lunch.
- *Compensatory Education.* Forty percent of elementary and secondary school children scoring at or below the twenty-fifth academic achievement percentile are served by Chapter 1 of the Education Consolidation and Improvement Act. Enrolled children score 15–20 percent better than comparable nonenrolled children in standardized reading and mathematics tests. Achievement gaps between African American and other elementary students are narrowed.
- *Education of Children with Disabilities.* The purpose of the Individuals with Disabilities Education Act is to assure that every child with a handicap aged 3 to 21 receives a free appropriate education in a nonrestrictive environment. This home- and community-based approach is associated with many personal gains as well as with a savings of two-thirds of a million dollars in lifetime institutionalization costs for some children.
- *Employment and Training.* The Job Training Partnership Act provides permanent authorization for job training programs serving youths. Evaluations document improvements in employability and wages.
- *Childhood Injury Prevention.* Injury is the leading cause of death for children after the first few months of life. Effective strategies for reducing injuries include compulsory seat belt restraints, upper-story window bars, bicycle safety helmets, product safety regulations, counseling during home visiting, and community media educational campaigns.
- *Lead Screening and Reduction.* As many as 20 percent of poor young children, especially urban minorities, have toxic levels of lead with resultant decreased intelligence, developmental delay, and behavior disorders. Screening of the environment and of children is the first step for preventive strategies. Fewer than half the states have active screening programs.
- *Smoking Cessation Programs for Pregnant Women.* Cigarette smoking during pregnancy, by about one-third of pregnant women, contributes more than any other determinant to low birthweight and other unfavorable outcomes. Participation in smoking cessation programs has been demonstrated to improve birthweights and reduce premature birth and infant deaths.

- *Home Visiting*. Home visiting to pregnant women and new mothers has been shown to improve participation in prenatal care, increase birthweight, enhance child development, reduce injuries, and reduce child abuse and neglect. Maternity-related home visiting is routine in most European countries but is rare in the United States except in circumscribed demonstration projects.

Expansion of the list of effective programs between 1985 and 1990 raises hope that the health of children improved over that period. Nevertheless, the record is checkered at best. The nation's experience with measles is a timely example. No new evaluations are required to demonstrate that measles immunizations are an effective preventive strategy. Indeed, speculations were strong in the late 1970s that the disease, as with smallpox, could be eradicated, and that objective was repeated in the health objectives for the nation for the year 2000.[6] The prospect is considerably dimmed, however, by the 16,236 cases of measles and the 41 resultant deaths reported in 1989.[7]

Experience and wisdom are sufficient to assure good health for many children now deprived of it.[8] Our nation's overwhelming failure of child health policy limits the impact of effective programs by not extending them to everyone who would benefit. We seem content to demonstrate program effectiveness and then to hope that in some unguided and underfinanced way other responsible parties—maybe communities or public-private interactions—will act on the wisdom displayed by successful demonstrations and will spontaneously replicate them wherever there is need. This does not much happen.

The Select Committee's list of effective programs is incomplete. Additions should include income supplementation, family planning, newborn screening, and well-child care. From this extended list I wish to discuss two programs—family planning and Head Start—because they incorporate elements from a number of the other specific interventions known to be effective. In both instances the benefits to family and child health are incontrovertible and the societal neglects from failure to extend benefits to families in need are longstanding. For both family planning and preschool child development programs, the experience of other countries provides important instruction for U.S. policy.

The Family Context

Conventional wisdom and the weight of research evidence combine to affirm that nurturing families provide the best—perhaps the essential—milieu for the favorable rearing of infants and children. No recent evidence is more compelling than Jessie Bierman's longitudinal study from the 1970s demonstrating that secure and stable families contribute substantially to the health and well-being of children.[9] Bierman and her colleagues found that among infants born with severe complications, predominantly low birthweight, the early disadvantages tended to wash away among children reared in households with favorable socioeconomic status, stable families, and skilled mothers. Conversely, nearly one-third of children whose physical and developmental examinations during infancy revealed no problems had acquired one or more by age ten. Children at extraordinary risk were those reared in poverty, in unstable families, or with mothers having low educational levels. The children's health and adjustment problems included learning disabilities, poor school achievement, physical abnormalities, and behavioral disturbances. Variations on Bierman's findings have been confirmed repeatedly in the intervening decades.[10] An ambitious study reported at the Cornell conference on health policy in 1990 confirmed that well-financed community interventions can assist families with high-risk newborns to achieve for them improved development and health outcomes.[11]

Recent changes in the social and economic characteristics of the U.S. family are profound and well known. High poverty rates in households with children, increase in single-parent families, dramatically rising divorce rates, increase in reconstructed families, and employment of both parents outside the home are commonly cited attributes that characterize the changing U.S. family. Another characteristic not so commonly considered is the increasing rate of unwanted childbearing. A social philosophy that impedes access to services for preventing and terminating unwanted pregnancies yields a harvest of unwanted children who may be beyond the redemptive power of usual family social supports and interventions.

Unwanted Childbearing

About 12 percent of childbearing in the United States is unwanted—about every eighth newborn. Another 27 percent of births are mistimed—wanted some time but not just now.[12] The trend in unwanted childbearing has been upward by about 29 percent since 1982, reversing a previous downward trend. Between 1973 and 1982, the proportion of unwanted births to ever-married women was reduced almost by half. (The 1973 data do not include unmarried women.) High rates and unfavorable trends in unwanted and mistimed childbearing are accentuated among vulnerable populations such as teenagers, poor people, minorities, or the unmarried, but the problem is not unique to these groups. Although ever-married women have a lower rate of unwanted childbearing, they nonetheless bear most of the unwanted births, and among these women, the majority are older than 24, currently married, and living at more than 150 percent of the poverty level.[13]

Social policies that contribute to trends in unwanted childbearing are not free of controversy, but they strongly suggest that ground gained in the 1970s enabling women to limit their fertility was lost in the 1980s. It was a time associated with a one-third reduction in public funding of contraceptive services, and reduced access to abortion.[14] These associations are compelling and raise additional questions. Do the inadequate financing and implementation of programs known to be effective for promoting child health represent a national policy that reinforces the unwantedness of children? To what extent do inadequate social and health supports impose a burdensome and unreasonable self-sufficiency on young parents and cause many women to construe unintended pregnancies as unwanted? To what extent do these troubling circumstances contribute to family dysfunction? Being unwanted or even unintended is an unpromising prospect for the nurture of infants and children.

Concern about high rates of unwanted childbearing leads directly to considerations of child health. The issues include infant homicide, the leading U.S. cause of death from injury for children younger than one year of age.[15] Abuse and neglect of children increased during the 1980s at a rate beyond any that can be attributed to heightened public attention and reporting.[16] More than 2 million reports of abuse and neglect are filed annually in the United States, representing about 3.4 percent of all U.S. children. Conventional wisdom supports a linkage between unwanted childbearing and abuse and neglect. The linkage is confirmed and quantified in a study demonstrating that a child from a family with two unplanned births is 2.8 times more likely to be abused than a child from a family with no unplanned births; one from a family with three unplanned births is 4.6 times more likely to be abused.[17]

Unwanted childbearing associates with indicators of poor pregnancy outcome: inadequate prenatal care, use of alcohol and cigarettes during pregnancy, and low birthweight.[18] So far as I know, studies are not available to confirm or quantify possible linkages between unwanted childbearing and participation in programs that promote child health, such as immunizations, WIC, EPSDT, and Head Start. Problems of inadequate access resulting from underfinancing plague all of these programs, but motivational factors associated with reluctant parenthood surely play a role contributing to low utilization rates.

Lessons from Western Europe in these respects are instructive. Where surveys of adolescent sexual behavior have been reported, the findings do not vary greatly from those in the United States.[19] Major differences pertain to contraceptive efficiency. U.S. couples are poor contraceptors when compared with European counterparts. As a consequence, the U.S. rates of unplanned pregnancies are strikingly higher than in Europe (e.g., United States, 36.9 percent; Netherlands, 7.8 percent; Great Britain, 21 percent).[20] U.S. fertility rates are reduced to levels comparable to Western Europe only because the U.S. abortion rate is one of the highest in the Western world. (Induced abortions per 100 pregnancies in the United States, 27.3; Netherlands, 5.3; Canada, 10. 2; Denmark, 18.3; England and Wales, 14.2; Norway, 16.8.)[21] Data from the Netherlands are notable: Few barriers exist either to contraception or abortion; and rates for unplanned pregnancy and for abortion are exceedingly low. Attitudinal differences also pertain. At a recent international conference on child health, the Dutch delegate was asked if adolescents in his country could obtain contraception without parental consent. He responded that of course they could but that in most families a parent assisted with the adolescent's visit for contraception as soon as it seemed developmentally appropriate.[22]

Tracking Preschool Children

In the United States a great deal of data are available about childbearing women and newborns, but not much is known about the health condition of very young children. Nearly all infants in the United States are attended at birth by health professionals who provide some level of health status assessment and screening. Infants and young children are not assured another heath evaluation until school enrollment, when school districts and most states require proof of immunization. In between these mooring points a great many children are at sea. Their developmental and health service needs are well studied, but no tracking or monitoring system assures their individual needs are met.

International comparisons of child health help focus new attention on preschool programs of child development.[23] Indicators of child health in Western Europe are more favorable than those in the United States. A number of these indicators relate to the preschool-age population: immunization rates for 2-year-olds, deaths from injury, abuse and neglect, participation in well-child care, and routine screening. Comparative analysis of programs serving this population reveals major national differences in the tracking and monitoring systems for preschoolers' health. In most Western European countries, young children are tracked from the time of birth to assure linkage with appropriate health-related services. Tracking is often facilitated by health visitors who make home visits on every newborn and who continue oversight to assure participation in appropriate services.[24] Other countries use an approach that is less labor intensive. In the Netherlands, the mother of every newborn is given a stack of computer cards designating the time and place for the infant's follow-up visits. Each card is surrendered when the designated visit is made. Failure of a card to appear at a central registry prompts follow-up visitation to assist the family with a rescheduled visit.[25] Whatever the method of tracking, it is supplemented within a few years by one attached either to a system of community child health clinics or to preschools.

Attendance at preschools by age 3 or 4 is nearly universal among Western European children.[26] Preschools are usually a voluntary downward extension of the compulsory primary and secondary educational systems. Out-of-pocket payment for attendance at preschools is negligible—often the cost of a lunch. Attendance is usually for part of a day, a circumstance made possible by the generally lower rate of employment among mothers of preschoolers in Europe and a higher rate of part-time employment among working mothers.[27] Routine preventive health services are usually rendered in the context of the preschool, thereby assuring early identification of children with special health care and educational needs.

The major U.S. programs concerned with early identification of children with special needs include Title V of the Social Security Act (the Maternal and Child Health Block Grant); the EPSDT component of Medicaid (Title XIX); Head Start; and the Education of the Handicapped Act Amendments of 1986, known as Public Law 99-457. These programs vary greatly in scale, purpose, and effectiveness. The oldest and least well financed is Title V. It has been modified many times over its fifty-year history. It currently helps support the maternal and child health activities sponsored by state and local health departments. As a result of conditions imposed by the Omnibus Reconciliation Act of 1989 the Title V agencies are acquiring increasing skills for needs assessment and for cooperative planning with WIC, Head Start, and EPSDT. The financial base for the programs is too small to enable effective implementation of these plans in most states.

EPSDT mandates that states provide Medicaid-eligible children with screening, diagnostic, and treatment services. The guidelines define one of the most complete preventive health services programs available for U.S. children. The program has been painfully slow and incomplete in its implementation. The authorization was passed by Congress in 1967; regulations were not issued until 1972, after litigation by advocacy groups to release impounded funds. Further court action was required in many states to initiate the program. Tensions concerning the roles for public and private providers have surrounded the program. Few communities have engaged in extensive eligible case-finding or in the establishment of linkage to providers sufficient for the needs of all eligible children. A 1990 analysis revealed that only 20 percent of Medicaid-eligible children received EPSDT services and that on average only 1.3 percent of state Medicaid benefits was spent on EPSDT.[28] Among those children who are screened, a high proportion is found to have health problems in need of further attention.

Public Law 99-457 provides federal funds to the states to plan for providing nondiscriminatory education and health services to infants and toddlers who are handicapped or at risk for developing handicapping conditions. By 1991 all states were expected to fully implement mandated services for children beginning at age 3 and by 1993 electively beginning at birth. Judgments about probable success are premature, but note can be made of many serious problems. Among them is the requirement that each state develop a comprehensive system of child-find to assure participation of every child in need. Tracking systems that identify potentially eligible children prenatally or neonatally are proposed, but no model is entirely adequate or presently functional.[29] The situation is reminiscent of earlier efforts in Western Europe to establish risk registries for children with potential need for more than routine health care. The registries were eventually abandoned because they listed a high proportion of children with no handicapping condition and omitted many children who later required special attentions. An alternative approach has been advanced by Richards and Roberts:

> The widespread adoption of the idea of an "at risk" register for the detection of handicapping diseases in infancy has led to a situation in which an undefined population is being screened for undefined conditions by people who, for the most part, are untrained to detect the conditions for which they are looking. The "at risk" concept is an unsound basis for the detection of handicapping disorders; there is no alternative to the clinical examination of all infants in the neonatal period, their screening for metabolic and auditory defects at the proper ages, and the careful observation of every infant's developmental progress by doctors, supported by health visitors.[30]

A Comprehensive Development Program

Head Start distinguishes itself among U.S. child health and development programs in a number of important ways. For those who are served, Head Start provides the most comprehensive and sustained developmental and health care program available for U.S. poverty-level children. The program was inaugurated with breathtaking speed. Late in 1964 a panel of pediatric and child development experts recommended to the Office of Economic Opportunity that preschool programs be implemented to help poor children develop to their full potential. The recommendation was authorized early the next year, and by the following summer 561,359 children were enrolled in 11,068 centers. The energetic professionalism of the administrator, Julius Richmond; the willingness of government to spend liberally on behalf of domestic programs; and the hustling zeal of a widespread community action infrastructure, newly established by the War on Poverty, all came together with expansive effectiveness.

The initial six weeks' screening enrollments were later extended, and the program was supplemented in many other important ways. The program has become a durable part of community life and national policy even as some of the circumstances contributing to its dramatic beginnings were profoundly changed. In the 25 years of Head Start's existence, more than 11 million children have been served, along with many of their parents and families. Few other public service programs have been so thoroughly researched for both long- and short-term effectiveness. For that reason alone the program deserves careful attention for lessons that might apply to other initiatives on behalf of children's health.

Head Start brings together four major components: health care, education, social services, and parental involvement. Zigler emphasizes that Head Start is not adequately characterized either as an educational or as a child care program—it is an amalgam of *developmentally appropriate services*.[31] The amalgam undergoes periodic revision. Working parents press for expansion of Head Start to full-day services. Some programs have done so, often with funds other than the Head Start grant. The Silver Ribbon Panel evaluating Head Start's 25-year performance made recommendations for the future including full-day programs for those in need.[32]

Evaluative findings of Head Start include the following:[33]

- Children enrolled in Head Start enjoy immediate gains in cognitive scores; these gains are not sustained in the long run.
- Program participants score higher than controls in self-esteem, achievement motivation, and social behavior after the first year; studies on the persistence of these advantages yield mixed results.
- Head Start centers facilitate meaningful improvement in children's health. Head Start children are more likely than non–Head Start enrollees to receive medical and dental examinations; speech, language, and developmental assessments; nutritional evaluations; metabolic, vision, and hearing screenings; adequate diets; and all appropriate immunizations.
- Close collaboration between Head Start programs and other community agencies is well established. Joint staff training with local school access occurs in 80 percent of the districts (1985 report); Head Start centers occupy public school buildings in 58 percent of the districts; and 20 percent of all Head Start programs are operated by school systems. (Other sponsors are community action agencies, 40 percent; private nonprofit corporations, 28 percent; and other groups, 12 percent.)

- Head Start families are diverse and have changed over the years. A sizable proportion is white, black, or Hispanic; a large proportion has only one parent at home; only about 50 percent of the household heads are working; about 30–40 percent of the mothers are working; and most households have three or four children.

The enduring benefits from participating in a comprehensive preschool developmental program are affirmed from other sources.[34] The Perry Preschool Project in Ypsilanti, Michigan, assigned a randomly selected group of 3- and 4-year-olds from low-income families to a high-quality preschool and to a control group. At age 19, members of the preschool group, as compared with the controls, were more likely to have graduated from high school, to be enrolled in postsecondary education, and to be employed and were less likely to have committed crimes, to be receiving welfare assistance, or to have borne children during the teen years. The long-range favorable impact of an intervention at ages 3 to 4 years is a stunning finding. It demonstrates that the destructive influence of poverty on child health and development can be ameliorated by modest interventions that fall far short of politically troublesome schemes to redistribute income—desirable as they may be.

The major disappointment of Head Start is its failure to reach for enrollment of more than 20 percent of eligible children. The constraint is in large part fiscal, a limitation Congress may correct by authorizing a $7 billion budget for 1994, which would be sufficient to serve all eligible 3-, 4-, and 5-year-olds. Recommendations for Head Start's future, proposed by the Silver Ribbon Panel, go even further. They include programs for children younger than 3 years and flexibility in income guidelines.[35] At the same time, the panel urged expansion of other federal programs critical to children and families. Part of Head Start's success requires linkage with other health and social support services and stimulation and expansion of those that are deficient. "Head Start cannot fill in the gaps for a system plagued by inadequate housing, health, and other family supports."[36]

Head Start helps demonstrate what circumstances can promote participation in comprehensive health care for young children. North identified the characteristics more than a decade ago:[37]

1. Health services are planned and administered through a school or school-like organization whose primary function is education and child development, not child health.
2. Personal health services are provided by a variety of physicians, dentists, clinics, and health workers already serving the communities in which Head Start centers are located. Only a minority of ser-

vices are provided in the centers or by full-time staff. Funds from a variety of sources are used to pay for such services.

3. The Head Start program provides each child and family with an advocate who does whatever is necessary to ensure that needed care is sought for the child and is actually provided when sought.

Proponents of essential primary care and preventive health services sometimes dilate on narrowly medicalized models. One example encompasses diagnostic, treatment, consultative, and referral services; diagnostic laboratory and radiologic services; emergency medical services; preventive dental services; transportation; and pharmaceutical services. The list goes on to include medical social services, immunizations, EPSDT, prenatal care, and blood pressure screening. Although young children should have access to this splendid array of expensive care, very few children will need and, if lucky, make use of all of it. The list misses by a long shot the kind of comprehensive care needed by most young children and their families. Head Start better defines their needs. The health care of very young children features parental counseling and support, developmental assessment and stimulation, and routine preventive health care, much of which can be rendered by nurses and other practitioners outside the domains of high-tech medicine. Developmental and preventive health care programs must also assure facilitation of linkage to more extensive social and medical services as appropriate. Head Start demonstrates that such linkages are feasible.

The Head Start/EPSDT combination would be a powerful entitlement to assure the healthful development of this country's children. It is a combination that could be implemented in most locales by some combination of community action agencies, schools, health departments, and community health centers, often with the help of private practitioners. As the nation contemplates health service reforms, these service elements deserve more attention and support than they now receive.

Some Lessons Learned

A Family Role in Children's Health

The composition of families is changing. Kahn and Kamerman required 16 different models to fully characterize U.S. families.[38] This diversity is sometimes regarded as evidence of the family's disintegration. It may instead be regarded as evidence of a diversity that liberates people, especially women, from stereotypic roles and from the depressive circumstances that confine many poverty-level mothers.[39] Families of widely diverse composition can raise healthy children. If given a supportive structure in which to assist the health and development of young children, as in Head Start, many parents will be responsive.[40] The experience of Head Start dispels the myth that community supports and services weaken families and contribute to their dependency. Those are the consequences of neglect. Children and families require help, and they respond constructively to it. The families of diverse composition who participate in Head Start raise children who are more self-sufficient, more productive, and less dysfunctional than children from nonparticipating families.

A Community Role in Children's Health

Initiative and strength reside, sometimes in latent forms, in nearly all communities. Many of them display these attributes from time to time,[41] and nearly all communities manifest initiative and strength when a serious national purpose stimulates, mobilizes, and provides the community with resources (e.g., community action agencies and Head Start). Child and family support systems are inexpensive when organized at the community level—but they are not bootstrap operations. Child health and family support services consistently available across place and time must be institutionalized in government as matters of high priority. The public responsibility does not diminish or deny substantial private or voluntary roles—but their variability and self-protective prerogatives need to be exercised within some broad public guarantees assured on behalf of all eligible people.

A Federal Role in Children's Health

Much constructive action on behalf of families and children can be initiated and can flourish under the authority of local and state governments. The history of Title V (the MCH Block grant) and Title XIX (Medicaid and EPSDT) demonstrate this to be true. Those histories also demonstrate that when broad discretion about program content and support is vested at local levels, many of them will opt for neglect. A strong federal role in defining standards, providing resources, and monitoring performance does not preclude substantial community involvement (e.g., Head Start, community health centers). In 1935, the Social Security Act did not establish old-age pensions and unemployment compensation as matters of local option. Likewise, we should not permit children's health and family support to be such options. Social interventions to improve children's health are not apt to be extensively implemented or successful without strong national leadership. Token programs, promises of demonstration projects, and upbeat exhortations delivered along with starvation programmatic rations will not serve the nation or its children.

Finally, we must establish beyond any doubt that children are wanted—both by their families and by the larger society. A society that neglects and fails its children, as ours does in so many ways, can scarcely expect parents to provide supportive nurture. A search for successful social interventions on behalf of children's health yields rich evidence about programs that work. What fails to work is indifference to that evidence. What will work is a mobilized national will to help children and their families. It should be an important part of any national program to reform systems of health care financing and access.

Notes

1. D. T. Ellwood, *Poor Support: Poverty in the American Family* (New York: Basic Books, 1988); and L. B. Schorr, *Within Our Reach: Breaking the Cycle of Disadvantage* (New York: Doubleday, 1988).

2. R. H. McKey, L. Condelli, H. Ganson et al., *The Impact of Head Start on Children, Families, and Communities*, DHHS Pub. No. (OHDS) 85–31193 (Washington, D.C.: Government Printing Office, 1985).

3. L. V. Klerman, *Alive and Well? A Research and Policy Review of Health Programs for Poor Young Children* (New York: National Center for Children in Poverty, School of Public Health, Columbia University, 1991).

4. Select Committee on Children, Youth, and Families, U.S. House of Representatives, *Opportunities for Success: Cost-Effective Programs for Children Update* (Washington, D.C.: Government Printing Office, 1990).

5. Select Committee, *Opportunities for Success*; and Klerman, *Alive and Well?*

6. U.S. Public Health Service, *Healthy People* 2000: National Health Promotion and Disease Prevention Objectives, DHHS Pub. No. (PHS) 91–50212 (Washington, D.C.: U.S. Public Health Service, 1991).

7. American Academy of Pediatrics, *Report of the Committee on Infectious Diseases* (Elk Grove, Ill.: American Academy of Pediatrics, 1991); and Public Health Service, *Healthy People* 2000.

8. Klerman, *Alive and Well?*

9. E. E. Werner, J. M. Bierman, and F. E. French, *The Children of Kauai* (Honolulu: University of Hawaii Press, 1971).

10. William T. Grant Foundation Commission on Work, Family, and Citizenship, *The Forgotten Half: Pathways to Success for America's Youth and Young Families* (Washington, D.C.: William Grant Foundation Commission, 1988).

11. The Infant Health and Development Program, "Enhancing the Outcomes of Low-Birth-Weight, Premature Infants: A Multisite, Randomized Trial," *Journal of the American Medical Association* 263(1990):3035–3042.

12. L. B. Williams and W. F. Pratt, "Wanted and Unwanted Childbearing in the U.S. 1973–88," *Advance Data*, National Center for Health Statistics 189(1990):1–8.

13. Williams and Pratt, "Wanted and Unwanted Childbearing."

14. R. B. Gold and D. Daley, "Public Funding of Contraceptive, Sterilization, and Abortion Service, Fiscal Year 1990," *Family Planning Perspectives* 23(1991): 204–211;

and S. K. Henshaw and J. Van Vort, "Abortion Services in the United States, 1987 and 1988," *Family Planning Perspectives* 22(1990):102–108, 142.

15. A. E. Waller, S. P. Baker, and A. Szocka, "Childhood Injury Deaths: National Analysis and Geographic Variations," *American Journal of Public Health* 79(1989):310–315.

16. Select Committee on Children, Youth, and Families, U.S. House of Representatives, *Abused Children in America: Victims of Official Neglect* (Washington, D.C.: Government Printing Office, 1987).

17. S. J. Zuravin, "Unplanned Childbearing and Family Size: Their Relationship to Child Neglect and Abuse," *Family Planning Perspectives* 23(1991):155–161.

18. National Center for Health Statistics, *Health Aspects of Pregnancy and Childbirth, United States* 1982, DHHS Pub. No. (PHS) 99–1992 (Hyattsville, Md.: U.S. Public Health Service, 1988).

19. E. F. Jones, J. D. Forrest, S. K. Henshaw et al., "Unintended Pregnancy, Contraceptive Practice, and Family Planning Services in Developed Countries," *Family Planning Perspectives* 20(1988):53–67.

20. Jones, Forrest, Henshaw et al., "Unintended Pregnancy."

21. S. K. Henshaw, "Induced Abortion: A World Review," *Family Planning Perspectives* 16(2)(1990):59–76.

22. H. P. Verbrugge, "Unrecorded Comment, Conference on Child Health in 1990: The U.S. Compared to Canada, England and Wales, France, the Netherlands, and Norway," *Pediatrics* 86(6, part 2)(1990).

23. B. C. Williams and C. A. Miller, *Preventive Health Care for Young Children: Findings from a* 10-Country Study and Directions for U.S. Policy (Arlington, Va.: National Center for Clinical Infant Programs, 1991).

24. S. Goodwin, "Child Health Services in England and Wales: An Overview," *Pediatrics* 86(6, part 2) (1990):1032–1036.

25. H. P. Verbrugge, "Youth Health Care in the Netherlands: A Bird's Eye View," *Pediatrics* 86(6, part 2) (1990):1044–1047.

26. W. Tietze and K. Ulferman, "An International Perspective on Schooling for 4-Year-Olds," *Theory into Practice* 28(1989):69–77.

27. P. Moss, "Childcare and Equality of Opportunity," *Consolidated Report to the European Commission* (Brussels: Commission of the European Communities, 1988).

28. I. T. Hill and J. M. Breyel, *Caring for Kids* (Washington, D.C.: National Governors' Association, 1991).

29. C. Berman, P. Biro, and E. S. Fenichel, *Keeping Track: Tracking Systems for High-Risk Infants and Young Children* (Arlington, Va.: National Center for Clinical Infant Programs, 1989).

30. D. G. Richards and C. J. Roberts, "The 'At Risk' Infant," *Lancet* 7518(2)(1967):711–713.

31. S. L. Kagan and E. F. Zigler, "Early Schooling: A National Opportunity?" in S. L. Kagan and E. F. Zigler, eds., *Early Schooling: The National Debate* (New Haven, Conn.: Yale University Press, 1987).

32. J. Lombardi, "Head Start: The Nation's Pride, a Nation's Challenge. Recommendations for Head Start in the 1990s," *Young Children* September(1990):22–29.

33. McKey et al., *The Impact of Head Start.*

34. P. P. Olmsted, "Early Childhood Care and Education in the United States. Chapter XV," in P. P. Olmsted and D. P. Weikart, eds., *How Nations Serve Young Children* (Ypsilanti, Mich.: High Scope Press, 1989).

35. Lombardi, "Head Start."

36. Lombardi, "Head Start."

37. F. North, Jr., "Health Services in Head Start," in *Project Head Start: A Legacy of the War on Poverty* (New York: Free Press, 1979).

38. A. J. Kahn and S. B. Kamerman, *Income Transfers for Families with Children: An Eight-Country Study* (Philadelphia: Temple University Press, 1983).

39. S. Orr and S. James, "Maternal Depression in an Urban Pediatric Practice: Implications for Health Care Delivery," *American Journal of Public Health* 74(1984):363–365.

40. R. K. Leik and M. A. Chalkley, "Parent Involvement: What Is It That Works?" *Children Today* 19(1990):34–37.

41. Schorr, *Within Our Reach.*

9

Health Care of the Poor: The Contribution of Social Insurance

Diane Rowland

Once again we are engaged as a nation in a policy debate over the shape of our health insurance system. With more than 30 million Americans without health insurance coverage and many others fearful that escalating costs will undermine their protection, the call for comprehensive reform to provide coverage to all Americans has become central to the debate over future directions for this nation.

As the debate moves forward, the difficult issues of how to divide public and private responsibility, who and what to cover, and how to finance this coverage must be addressed in the fashioning of a better policy. Intrinsic to these discussions of broadening health coverage are the related issues of how to finance care for the poor and whether to provide such coverage under a universal social insurance approach or a more targeted and income-tested approach. Lessons drawn from the Medicare and Medicaid experience provide insights into the implications of these two models for care of the poor under national health care reform.

Medicaid is our nation's health care financing program for the poor, serving one in ten Americans. It is a means-tested and targeted program designed for the welfare population and intended only for those with limited income and resources. As the federal government's partner in Medicaid's provision of care to the poor, states both administer the program and provide up to half of the financing. Medicare, in contrast, operates as a

This chapter was prepared with support from the Henry J. Kaiser Family Foundation. The views reflected in the paper do not necessarily represent those of the Kaiser Foundation, the Kaiser Commission of the Future of Medicaid, or Johns Hopkins University. The author gratefully acknowledges the helpful comments and assistance of Judy Feder and Liz Fowler in the preparation of this chapter.

fully federal program providing nearly universal coverage for Americans age 65 and older and for those with permanent and total disabilities. The scope of benefits under Medicare does not vary by income or geographic residence and remains essentially as enacted in 1965.

This chapter examines the link between health care of the poor and social insurance through an assessment of the Medicare and Medicaid models. The impact of Medicaid, as the primary insurer for the nonelderly poor, and of Medicare, as the insurer of the elderly, on the health of the poor and access to care provides valuable lessons for national health care reform.

Medicaid and Health Care of the Poor

In the years preceding Medicaid's enactment, the financing and provision of health care to the poor was a meager combination of charity care and reliance on public hospitals and clinics coupled with limited public welfare–based assistance. Medicaid was intended to reform the financing of care to the poor by providing grants to states for the care of the medically indigent. From its enactment in 1965, Medicaid notably reshaped health care for the poor in the United States.

The Pre-Medicaid Environment

The Social Security Act of 1935 set up the nation's retirement benefit and unemployment insurance system. It also established the nation's welfare system to provide cash payments to the aged, the blind, and single-parent families with dependent children. The categories of individuals eligible for public assistance reflected the concept of "deserving poor" embodied in the Elizabethan poor laws of the seventeenth century.[1] As a result, many of the poor were ineligible for welfare assistance because they did not fall into a category eligible for aid.

Under the welfare system, the federal government provided funds to match 50 percent of state expenditures on behalf of the indigent who qualified for assistance. States set income eligibility levels and required near destitution before providing assistance. Direct financing of medical services was not permitted in the initial legislation, but states could include additional funds in cash benefit payments to welfare recipients to help cover the cost of medical care.[2]

The Social Security Act Amendments of 1950 broadened the states' authority by permitting direct vendor payments to providers for medical care for welfare recipients. The Kerr-Mills program of 1960 further broadened federal involvement in the medical care of the welfare poor by providing open-ended federal matching to the states for a specified set of medical services and coverage of the medically indigent aged.[3] Despite these expansions, medical vendor payments for welfare recipients remained inadequate and provided aid only to a small portion of the poverty population.[4]

Both the poor receiving welfare assistance and those without aid depended on charity care or public hospitals and clinics for medical care. State and local appropriations supported the public system, which was separate from the private facilities used by higher income and insured Americans. Patients who could pay for treatment received care from private practitioners in their medical offices, while patients who were poor received care through charity or local welfare departments. In the inner city, the poor often relied on the clinics of large teaching hospitals as their primary care provider.[5]

In the days before enactment of Medicaid, the poor were subjected to long waits in crowded hospital waiting rooms to obtain care and when hospitalized, were placed in charity wards or in the public hospital. Financial hardship and devastation were often associated with the need for medical care.[6] During this time, before the major civil rights legislation of the 1960s, segregation by health facilities and by practitioners further restricted access to care for poor minorities. Care of the poor was outside the mainstream of U.S. medical care.

The difficulties associated with receipt of care resulted in fewer services provided to the poor than to the nonpoor, despite the former's lower health status.[7] In a seminal work in the 1930s, the Committee on the Cost of Medical Care documented substantial disparities in the use of hospital and physician services between the poor and the upper-income population.[8] By the 1960s, little progress had been made to remedy these disparities.

Intentions and Impact of Medicaid

Medicaid was enacted in 1965 as companion legislation to the Medicare program to provide grants to states for medical assistance to the poor welfare population and the medically indigent who met the welfare categories. The concept of federal matching grants to the states for care of the medically indigent aged embodied in the 1960 Kerr-Mills legislation became the framework of Medicaid.

Medicaid is a joint federal-state program to provide health care to recipients of welfare assistance (Aid to Families with Dependent Children and Supplemental Security Income) and other needy individuals. The federal government provides matching grants to states for expenditures for covered services on behalf of eligible groups of people. Welfare standards and eligibility categories shape Medicaid's core eligibility rules. Federal guidelines place requirements on states for coverage of specific eligibility groups and benefits and give states the option to cover others. Within federal guidelines, states determine who will be covered, what services will be paid for, how much providers will be paid, and how the program will be administered.

The major goals of the Medicaid program were to ensure that those eligible for services received adequate care and to reduce the burden of medical care for those with limited financial resources.[9] This meant both the reduction or elimination of service use differentials between the poor and nonpoor and the elimination of the two-class medical care system.[10] By providing the poor with the financial ability to use private hospitals and doctors, Medicaid sought to broaden access to the "mainstream of medical care" and reduce reliance on charity care and the public system.

Access Differentials. Before the enactment of Medicaid, the poor were sicker than those with higher incomes but were less likely to receive medical care.[11] In 1964, the poor averaged 3. 8 physician visits per year compared to 4.7 visits for the nonpoor and 179 hospitalizations per 1, 000 compared to 202 hospitalizations per 1,000 for the nonpoor.[12] After the enactment of Medicaid, steady progress in reversing these access differentials occurred.

Studies of physician and hospital utilization by the poor found that by the 1980s, the poor no longer lagged behind the nonpoor in overall use of physician and hospital services and in some cases rates for the poor exceeded those of the nonpoor.[13] By 1978, the poor had an average of 6.2 physician visits per year and 297 hospitalizations per 1,000 compared to 5.0 visits and 239 hospitalizations per 1, 000 among the nonpoor.[14]

While showing dramatic progress in reversing the previous differentials between the poor and nonpoor, these statistics fail to account for the lower health status of the poor, which would be expected to result in more medical care use by the poor than the nonpoor.[15] When utilization is adjusted for health status, differences in use of ambulatory care between the poor and nonpoor persist, with the poor experiencing fewer visits than those with higher incomes.[16]

Comparisons of utilization levels of the poor and nonpoor are indicative of progress in improving access to care, but they do not provide a full measure of Medicaid's impact because they obscure differences in Medicaid coverage of the poor. More than half of the people living in poverty are not covered by Medicaid because they do not meet the income and categorical requirements for eligibility.[17] A more meaningful test of Medicaid's impact on access to care for the poor is provided by examining use of services for the poor with and without Medicaid coverage.

Analysis of utilization levels within the poverty population that controls for health status reveals striking differentials and shows that Medicaid coverage plays a significant role in reducing barriers to access to care.

The poor without Medicaid continue to lag significantly behind those with Medicaid or private insurance, whereas those with Medicaid use health services at the same rate as the nonpoor in similar health status.[18]

The poor without Medicaid averaged 3.9 physician contacts per year compared to 5.7 visits for the poor with Medicaid and 5.3 visits for the nonpoor population.[19] Among low-income children, the uninsured were less likely to see a physician and averaged 1 less visit per year than children with Medicaid or private insurance.[20] Among the poor who were sick, the uninsured used half the number of physician services as those with Medicaid coverage.[21]

Beyond improving use of services, Medicaid helps reduce the financial stress resulting from medical expenditures. Out-of-pocket expenditures for children as a percent of family income were fifteen times greater in families below the poverty level without Medicaid coverage as in comparable families with Medicaid.[22] The poor with Medicaid coverage had lower out-of-pocket expenses for medical care than the poor who were uninsured and were more likely to use dental services and prescription drugs in addition to physician and hospital care.[23] Medicaid coverage appears to help provide access to a broader service package that supplements physician care.

More recent studies have begun to raise questions, however, about the extent to which equality in utilization rates reflects equal care. A California study of sick newborns found that Medicaid and uninsured newborns had more severe health problems than privately insured newborns yet received fewer inpatient services.[24] Resources provided to the infants covered under Medicaid exceeded the services to the uninsured but were lower than the care levels provided to privately insured newborns. Other studies of the privately insured and uninsured adult population have found similar differences in hospital resource allocation and outcomes that favor the insured.[25]

Examination of Medicaid's impact on a national basis also obscures the significant variations that occur among the states in scope of coverage and accessibility to medical care. Low-income people receive less care from physicians if they reside in states with limited Medicaid programs.[26] Among Medicaid beneficiaries, the average number of visits to physicians is lower for those residing in states with restrictive coverage and limits on benefits than for those in states with more generous benefits.[27]

Mainstream Medical Care. Medicaid was intended to bring the poor into the mainstream of medical care by opening the private marketplace and expanding the range of providers willing to treat the poor.[28] Although concerns continue to be raised about the level of access of Medicaid patients to private physicians, Medicaid financing has clearly helped move care of the poor more into the mainstream.

For the poor with Medicaid, dependence on charity and free care has been replaced with financial access to both public and private providers. Hospitals are prohibited from discriminating against Medicaid patients, and Medicaid beneficiaries receive care from all types of hospitals. Medicaid continues to represent a higher proportion of the patient distribution in public hospitals, but Medicaid caseloads in both proprietary and nonprofit hospitals reflect broad access.[29] In contrast, care of the uninsured reflects a less equitable distribution, with proprietary hospitals having a lower proportion of uninsured patients and large teaching and public hospitals carrying a heavier responsibility than most nonprofit hospitals.

The poor who are uninsured are more reliant on free and public sources of care than are those with Medicaid coverage. In 1977, 20 percent of ambulatory physician visits for the uninsured poor in contrast to 5 percent for the poor with Medicaid reflected care from community health centers, state and local government, or charity care.[30] The uninsured poor are also more dependent on the availability of public hospital services for care, and in periods of Medicaid cutbacks such facilities may have inadequate resources to meet increased demand for care.[31]

Although access to care in private physicians' offices is an area where Medicaid has made progress, these attempts have clearly fallen short. The poor are less likely than the nonpoor to receive care from a physician in his or her office or by telephone contact.[32] Although 85 percent of Medicaid beneficiaries report a usual source of care, a rate comparable to that of the privately insured and notably higher than that of the uninsured, they are more likely than the privately insured to list a hospital outpatient department or emergency room as their usual source of care.[33] Fifty-six percent of nonelderly Medicaid beneficiaries report a physician's office as their usual source of care compared to 70 percent of privately insured patients.

Access to prenatal care is better for those with Medicaid than for the uninsured, but access to private physicians is still limited. Seventy-six (76 percent) of all pregnant women compared to 39 percent of pregnant women with Medicaid and 22 percent of poor pregnant women without any health care coverage receive prenatal care from private physicians.[34] Thirty-three percent of women with Medicaid and more than 50 percent of uninsured women rely on health departments and public sources for their care.

Provider participation in the Medicaid program has been a consistent problem in attempts to integrate Medicaid patients into the mainstream of ambulatory care. Many physicians either do not accept Medicaid patients or limit the extent of their Medicaid practice.[35] More than a quarter of physicians do not participate in the program at all.[36]

Low payment rates coupled with the administrative burden and liability concerns associated with Medicaid patients are frequently cited by physicians as reasons for nonparticipation in the program. Medicaid payment rates for physician services are considerably lower for comparable procedures than Medicare rates and most private fees.[37] A recent study found that Medicaid payments for pediatric care averaged less than two-thirds of private fees.[38]

Low payment levels appear to undermine Medicaid's ability to assure access to mainstream medical care for the Medicaid population. Although beneficiaries in high- and low-fee states appear to receive the same number of medical services, the site of care is less likely to be a physician's office in low-fee states.[39] Medicaid beneficiaries in high-fee states are more likely to receive care in physician's offices, while their counterparts in low-fee states obtain services in settings such as hospital outpatient departments and emergency rooms.

Health Status. The impact of Medicaid coverage on the health status of the poor is far more difficult to assess because direct causal links between the financing and availability of care and health outcomes have not been established. Most studies have examined differences in utilization of services and not addressed the more difficult measure of differences in outcome. Assessing outcomes is further complicated by the lack of income data in mortality and morbidity statistics.

It is clear, however, that following enactment of Medicaid, significant improvements in the health of the poor occurred with the greatest progress in death rates from causes that are traditionally higher among the poor and that are amenable to improved health care. Substantial declines were seen in infant and maternal mortality and death rates for major diseases, including diabetes and influenza and pneumonia.[40] Some achievements are attributable to improvements in medical treatment, sanitation, nutrition, and housing, but expanded availability of care through Medicaid has undoubtedly played a role.

Although the linkage between improved financing and use of medical care under Medicaid and improved health outcomes for the poor is primarily an associative relationship, use of medical care has been found to result in significantly lower mortality rates.[41] Most notably, results have shown that states covering first-time pregnancies under Medicaid have lower neonatal mortality rates than states that do not offer coverage.

What is more clearly documented is that the loss of Medicaid coverage and the absence of insurance can adversely affect health status. The termination of Medicaid coverage for chronically ill and poor adults in California was shown to result in decreased access to care, decreased satisfaction with the health system, and worsened health status.[42] Lack of insurance was shown to be associated with an elevated and increased risk of adverse outcome in newborns.[43] After controlling for the severity of the illness, comparisons of hospitalized patients found that those who were uninsured had a higher mortality risk than those with private insurance.[44]

Lessons from the Medicaid Experience

Medicaid has achieved significant advances in health care of the poor but has fallen short of realizing equity of access between the poor and nonpoor. Most notably, Medicaid's impact on overall care for the poor is limited because half of the poverty population is outside of Medicaid's welfare-based reach and because coverage varies across states. Progress in eliminating access differentials between the poor with Medicaid and the nonpoor has been remarkable, but this progress has been uneven across the states and has left the uninsured poor behind.

Medicaid is a means-tested program for individuals who fit the welfare-based categories of assistance and meet state-determined income and assets tests for eligibility. It is not designed to provide social insurance to the entire poverty population. Single individuals and childless couples as well as most two-parent families are excluded from coverage, no matter how poor. Once enrolled, coverage is dependent on the individual's continuing to meet income eligibility standards, which results in high turnover of the covered population. Many who are eligible for the program do not enroll because they are unwilling to apply to a welfare program or are turned away by procedural and informational barriers to enrollment. In essence, Medicaid is not a "user-friendly" program.

Concerns about access to mainstream medical care have remained throughout Medicaid's history. Physician participation has been a persistent problem undermining the goals of access to mainstream medical care. The poor, even those with Medicaid coverage, still rely much more heavily on the outpatient departments of hospitals and emergency rooms and clinics for their care than do those with private insurance. Fragmentation of care and episodic treatment are still targets for improvement in care to the poor.

The state-based nature of the program has also resulted in variations in coverage and benefits across the states. Medicaid is not a universal national program but rather a state-designed and implemented program that operates within federal guidelines. Program benefits and scope of coverage of the poor thus vary widely by state.[45] Access to health care services and the level of services largely depend on the state of residence and the scope of the Medicaid program in that state.[46]

The implementation of Medicaid has shown a program assuming growing responsibility for financing health services for the poor but constantly struggling with rising costs.[47] Concerns over escalating program costs resulted in the 1972 repeal of the provision in the original law requiring Medicaid to be comprehensive in scope of services and eligibility for welfare-covered groups by 1975.[48] Throughout its 25-year history, Medicaid has been subjected to cutbacks made in response to fiscal pressure in the states and concern over increasing program costs.[49] Cutbacks in recent years have eroded Medicaid coverage of the poor and have begun to reverse the progress in closing gaps in access to care across income groups.[50]

Medicaid as a program for the poor has enjoyed neither popular support nor a strong political constituency. It has come under attack from the poor as an inadequate insurer and from state and federal bill payers as a costly and growing share of the budget. The program's welfare base has left Medicaid with a weak political constituency and a vulnerability to cutbacks and retrenchment.[51] The program has had few allies and proponents, yet it survives because of its critical role in financing indigent care.

Medicare and Health Care of the Elderly Poor

When Medicare was enacted, 5 million elderly people representing 29 percent of the elderly population lived in poverty.[52] The plight of the elderly poor was a pressing national concern that led to improvements in medical assistance for elderly welfare recipients and to calls for broader reforms to provide medical care for all elderly people. Medicare, a new federal program establishing universal coverage for basic physician and hospital services, emerged from the debate. It was intended to provide all beneficiaries of Social Security with medical security to complement their retirement benefits.

The Pre-Medicare Environment

The 1963 Social Security Survey of the Aged documented that about half of all elderly people had no health insurance.[53] Private insurers were reluctant to offer policies to older people and most employers dropped coverage at retirement. Companies were reluctant to write individual policies for elderly people for fear of insuring an excessive number of poor risks. The available policies often limited coverage, exempted preexisting conditions, and in general offered inadequate protection.[54]

For the elderly poor, public assistance was limited. Under public welfare programs operated by the states with matching funds from the federal government, the elderly poor could receive some cash assistance and limited payment for medical care. In 1960, the Kerr-Mills program (Medical Aid to the Aged) expanded medical coverage under state-based welfare programs to include federal matching payments for the medically indigent aged with incomes slightly above the welfare levels.

In general, state welfare assistance for the elderly poor was more generous than that afforded to poor children and families. Nonetheless, indigent elderly people were dependent on the same system of public hospitals and clinics and charity care as the nonaged poor were. Access to care from the public sector entailed long waits and crowded conditions. The expense of care from private physicians was beyond the means of the impoverished elderly and a serious financial strain for others.[55]

Intentions and Impact of Medicare

Medicare was the culmination of a long struggle to improve financing of health care for the elderly. Medicare provides hospital and medical care insurance to Americans age 65 and older who are eligible for Social Security or Railroad Retirement benefits as well as to Americans who are permanently disabled. As a result, the federally administered Medicare program provides almost all elderly people with universal health insurance coverage irrespective of income or place of residence. Benefits and eligibility are uniform throughout the country.

Medicare is a social insurance program with the hospital component financed by payroll tax contributions of employers and employees and the physician component financed by premium payments by beneficiaries and general tax revenues. The Medicare program covers hospital care, limited posthospital skilled nursing facility care, physician services, outpatient hospital care, home health care, and some ambulatory services. Medicare does not cover prescription drugs, dental care, vision services, or long-term care. Medicare requires beneficiaries to pay a deductible for hospital and physician care as well as 20 percent co-insurance on physician services.

Medicare was intended both to improve access to care for the poor and nonpoor elderly and lighten the financial burden for medical services faced by the elderly.[56] Although the primary objective of Medicare was to protect the elderly against the possibility of large medical outlays, the program was also concerned with eliminating the financial barriers that discourage the elderly from seeking medical care and result in differential access to care.[57] Using Medicare provider participation to accomplish civil rights objectives was a part of the strategy to expand access.

Access Differentials. Access to health care services among the elderly population expanded significantly after the implementation of Medicare.[58] The percentage of elderly people seeking physician care and the number of physician visits increased substantially over pre-Medicare levels.[59] Use of hospital services also increased notably in the early years of the program and then leveled off in the 1970s.[60]

In expanding access for the full elderly population, Medicare appears to have been instrumental in reducing gaps in access to hospital and physician care for the elderly poor, minorities, and residents of rural areas. Prior to Medicare, the use of health services declined at lower income levels among the elderly. Early data following implementation of the program showed that these differentials persisted, with greater service use by the higher income elderly after health status differences had been taken into account.[61] By the late 1970s, the influence of income on health services use was removed among Medicare beneficiaries, although limited differences by race and residence persisted.[62]

For some of the low-income elderly, Medicaid serves as a supplement to Medicare by paying Medicare's cost sharing and premiums as well as augmenting Medicare benefits. Shortly after implementation of Medicare, an investigation of patterns of use of physician and hospital care among the elderly by income and health status found that the poor elderly with Medicaid coverage used services at rates commensurate with the middle-class elderly, whereas the poor elderly without Medicaid lagged considerably behind.[63] These differences by income and insurance status appeared to have been eliminated as the Medicare program matured. Analysis of utilization of ambulatory care services in 1982 revealed no statistically significant differences in the use of physician services between the elderly poor with or without Medicaid coverage and the elderly nonpoor.[64]

Medicare thus appears to have successfully eliminated differentials in access to health services by income. The experience of the elderly poor with universal Medicare coverage contrasts sharply with that of the nonelderly poor with Medicaid coverage, which varies by state. The nonelderly poor with Medicaid who reside in states with less generous coverage have lower physician use rates than the nonelderly poor with Medicaid coverage in more generous states. These differentials do not occur among the elderly poor, who have comparable access to care regardless of residence.[65]

Differentials in access to care within the elderly population appear to relate more to the adequacy of insurance coverage than to income. Lack of supplementary coverage from Medicaid or private insurance to help meet Medicare's cost-sharing obligations influences access to health care services by elderly people. An examination of ambulatory services utilization, controlling for socioeconomic and health status differences, shows that those relying solely on Medicare for coverage use fewer health services than those with supplementary coverage from either Medicaid or private insurance.[66] Elderly people with Medicare-only coverage are twice as likely to have no physician visits during a year as those with supplemental coverage, and those who use physician services incur fewer visits.

Financial Burden. Medicare has met with less success in achieving the objective of relieving the financial burden for medical care, especially among the low-income elderly. Medicare provides universal coverage to the elderly but also requires substantial cost sharing that is not income related and can be onerous.[67]

Gaps in Medicare coverage coupled with limits in the reach of Medicaid result in out-of-pocket payments that can be financially devastating for poor and near-poor elderly people living on limited and fixed incomes. On average, low-income elderly people spend 14 percent of their per capita income on out-of-pocket costs in contrast to 7 percent for higher-income elderly.[68] More than 33 percent of low-income elderly people incur catastrophic costs for medical care of more than 15 percent of their income compared to 6 percent of the nonpoor elderly. When hospitalized, 56 percent of the elderly with incomes of less than $10,000 a year experience catastrophic expenses.

Private supplementary insurance helps alleviate financial burdens by covering the hospital deductible and cost-sharing obligations under Medicare. Sixty-eight percent of the elderly have private insurance to protect against Medicare's cost-sharing requirements, but these policies are often not available or are too costly for the nearly 12 million elderly people with low incomes.[69] Medicaid is intended to fill the supplementary insurance role for low-income elderly people by paying Medicare cost sharing and providing additional services and payment of Medicare premiums. Medicaid offers important protection and helps improve the adequacy of Medicare coverage to the low-income elderly.

Medicaid, however, provides limited help to the elderly poor. Restrictive income and assets levels for eligibility under Medicaid and state variations in coverage leave 66 percent of the elderly poor and 90 percent of the near-poor without Medicaid assistance.[70] Recent legislation has extended eligibility to 120 percent of the poverty level, but the scope of coverage of the poor and near-poor varies. Moreover, many potentially eligible poor and near-poor elderly people do not obtain Medicaid assistance either from lack of knowledge about the program or reluctance to apply for "welfare" benefits.

Twenty-nine percent of the elderly poor have Medicaid coverage to supplement Medicare. Thirty-three percent of the elderly poor have Medicare coverage supplemented by private insurance, 33 percent rely solely on Medicare, and 3 percent are uninsured.[71] The elderly who rely solely on Medicare and the uninsured without Medicaid bear a far greater economic burden for health care services than do those with Medicaid. Nearly 70 percent of those without Medicaid spend more than 15 percent of their income on medical expenses compared to 25 percent of those with Medicaid coverage.[72]

Lessons from the Medicare Experience

The twenty-five years of health care coverage of the elderly by Medicare document the advantages of a universal program with a broad-based constituency. Universal eligibility for virtually all Americans over age 65 assures basic coverage across the elderly population and removes the fear of being uninsured that so many nonelderly people face. Enrollment in Medicare along with Social Security benefits is perceived as an earned right. All beneficiaries participate in the program without the stigma of public assistance faced by the Medicaid population.

For the elderly poor, Medicare has eliminated the two-class medical system and the heavy reliance on charity care in the years prior to Medicare's enactment. Examination of care patterns of Medicare beneficiaries shows broad access to a full range of health providers and facilities irrespective of income or race. In setting certification standards for program participation, Medicare served as a lever to accomplish racial desegregation and improve the quality of health facilities.

Essentially, Medicare has put an end to concern about differential access and discrimination in medical care of the elderly. Medicare has sought to restrain spending by containing payments to providers, yet such spending limits have not undermined access for Medicare beneficiaries as they appear to have for Medicaid beneficiaries. Medicare has both a larger market share than the welfare-linked Medicaid program and broader support.

For the most part, Medicare is a politically popular and protected program. From its enactment in 1965 through today, Medicare has remained basically the same in structure, scope, and benefits. Because Medicare covers almost all elderly people and is based on contributions during working years to support benefits in retirement, it is viewed as an earned right and social contract between government and retired workers. Medicare beneficiaries represent one of the most forceful voter constituencies in numbers and effectiveness.

From the perspective of the elderly poor, the fundamental strength of Medicare is that it brought equal benefits to all the elderly in one politically stable and uniform program. The fundamental flaw of Medicare is that it requires substantial out-of-pocket payments in conjunction with those uniform benefits. The financial burden of cost sharing hits those with low incomes hardest and requires supplementary assistance from programs such as Medicaid to moderate the fiscal strain. In the absence of subsidies or supplementation for the low-income population, Medicare shows that equal benefits with substantial cost sharing can disadvantage the elderly poor.[73]

Implications for National Health Care Reform

Medicare and Medicaid clearly were enacted with similar goals for the populations they served: improved access to care and reduced financial burden. In many ways, Medicare and Medicaid reflect a common success story as revealed by the dramatic improvements in access to care for the poor served by both programs. Most notably, differentials in use of hospital and physician services for the nonelderly poor with Medicaid and the elderly poor with Medicare in contrast to the comparable nonpoor population have been eliminated over the past 25 years.

The experiences of Medicaid and Medicare demonstrate that financing for health care services is a critical component in overcoming barriers to access to care. Although difficult to measure fully, better access resulting in more medical care has been shown to contribute to lower mortality rates and improved health. Without access to medical care, health suffers. Without medical insurance, the poor will continue to lag behind the nonpoor in access to medical services as well as health status. The nonelderly poor with Medicaid coverage fare better in obtaining health care services than do the poor who are uninsured, whereas the elderly poor on Medicare use services at rates comparable to higher-income elderly people.

When examining the differences between the universal social insurance approach of Medicare and the targeted means-tested approach of Medicaid, we can see that the Medicare model offers more positive results in improving access and integrating the poor into the mainstream of medical care than the Medicaid model. The universal coverage to all elderly people by Medicare assures full program participation by beneficiaries and provides a broad and powerful constituency to ensure that the program benefits are maintained and improved. The means-tested and state-financed Medicaid program has been vulnerable to cutbacks and constant attack. Medicare's uniform benefits and federal standards assure equity across states, whereas state discretion in shaping Medicaid has resulted in extensive variability in coverage and scope of benefits for the nonelderly poor.

Lessons from the two programs underscore the importance of universal financing with adequate benefits and protection for the poor in national health reform. From the Medicaid experience, we see the importance of uniform benefits and integration of the poor into a broader program with stronger political support and security. From the experience of Medicare, we see the importance in a universal program of making sure that cost sharing does not serve to erode the adequacy of benefits or create financial barriers to care for modest- and low-income people.

Notes

1. R. Stevens and R. Stevens, *Welfare Medicine in America: A Case Study of Medicaid* (New York: Free Press, 1974), pp. 19–56.

2. Stevens and Stevens, *Welfare Medicine in America.*

3. K. Davis and C. Schoen, "Health, Use of Medical Care, and Income," in *Health and the War on Poverty: A Ten-Year Appraisal* (Washington, D.C.: Brookings Institution, 1976), pp. 18–48.

4. Stevens and Stevens, *Welfare Medicine in America.*

5. E. R. Brown, "Medicare and Medicaid: The Process, Value and Limits of Health Care Reforms," *Journal of Public Health Policy* (September 1983): 335–356.

6. K. Davis, "Achievements and Problems of Medicaid," *Public Health Reports* (Washington, D.C.: U.S. Department of Health, Education, and Welfare)91(July–August 1976), pp. 309–316.

7. Davis and Schoen, "Health, Use of Medical Care, and Income," pp. 18–49.

8. Brown, "Medicare and Medicaid," pp. 335–356.

9. Davis and Schoen, "Health, Use of Medical Care, and Income," pp. 18–49.

10. Stevens and Stevens, *Welfare Medicine in America*; Brown, "Medicare and Medicaid," pp. 335–356.

11. Davis and Schoen, "Health, Use of Medical Care, and Income," pp. 18–49.

12. D. Rogers, R. Blendon, and T. Moloney, "Who Needs Medicaid?" *New England Journal of Medicine* 307(July 1, 1982):13–18.

13. K. Davis and R. Reynolds, "The Impact of Medicare and Medicaid on Access to Medical Care," in R. N. Rosset, ed., *The Role of Health Insurance in the Health Services Sector* (Washington, D.C.: Brookings Institution, 1977), pp. 391–425; R. W. Wilson and E. L. White, "Changes in Morbidity, Disability, and Utilization Differentials Between the Poor and the Nonpoor: Data from the Health Interview Survey: 1964 and 1973," *Medical Care* 15(August 1977): 636–646; P. Newacheck, "Access to Ambulatory Care for Poor Persons," *Health Services Research* 23(August 1988):401–419; Rogers, Blendon, and Moloney, "Who Needs Medicaid?" pp. 13–18; K. Davis, "Achievements and Problems of Medicaid," pp. 309–316.

14. Rogers, Blendon, and Moloney, "Who Needs Medicaid?" pp. 13–18.

15. J. Kaspar, "Health Status and Utilization: Differences by Medicaid Coverage and Income," *Health Care Financing Review* 7(1986):1–17; P. Newacheck and B. Starfield, "Morbidity and Use of Ambulatory Care Services Among Poor and Non-Poor Children," *American Journal of Public Health* 78(1988):927–935.

16. J. Kleinman, M. Gold, and D. Makuc, "Use of Ambulatory Medical Care by the Poor: Another Look at Equity," *Medical Care* 19(October 1981):1011–1029; Davis and Reynolds, "The Impact of Medicare and Medicaid on Access to Medical Care," pp. 391–425; Newacheck, "Access to Ambulatory Care for Poor Persons," pp. 401–419; Davis, "Achievements and Problems of Medicaid," pp. 309–316.

17. E. M. Howell, "Low Income Persons' Access to Health Care: NMCUES Medicaid Data," *Public Health Reports* 103(1988): 507–516.

18. G. R. Wilensky and M. L. Berk, "Health Care, the Poor and the Role of Medicaid," *Health Affairs* (1982):93–106; M. Rosenbach, "The Impact of Medicaid on Physician Use by Low-Income Children," *American Journal of Public Health* 79(Septem-

ber 1989):1220–1226; Davis and Reynolds, "The Impact of Medicare and Medicaid on Access to Medical Care," pp. 391–425; Howell, "Low Income Persons' Access to Health Care," pp. 507–516; Newacheck, "Access to Ambulatory Care for Poor Persons," pp. 401–419.

19. Newacheck, "Access to Ambulatory Care for Poor Persons," pp. 401–419.

20. Rosenbach, "The Impact of Medicaid on Physician Use by Low-Income Children," pp. 1220–1226.

21. Wilensky and Berk, "Health Care, the Poor and the Role of Medicaid," pp. 93–106.

22. P. Newacheck and N. H. Halfon, "The Financial Burden of Medical Care Expenses for Children," *Medical Care* 241(December 1986):1110–1117.

23. Wilensky and Berk, "Health Care, the Poor and the Role of Medicaid," pp. 93–106.

24. P. Braveman, S. Egerter, T. Bennett, and J. Showstack, "Differences in Hospital Resource Allocation Among Sick Newborns According to Insurance Coverage," *Journal of the American Medical Association* 266(December 18, 1991):3300–3308.

25. J. Hadley, E. Steinberg, and J. Feder, "Comparison of Uninsured and Privately Insured Hospital Patients," *Journal of the American Medical Association* 265(January 16, 1991):374–379.

26. R. Blendon, L. Aiken, H. Freeman, B. Kirkman-Liff, and J. Murphy, "Uncompensated Care by Hospitals or Public Insurance for the Poor: Does It Make a Difference?" *New England Journal of Medicine* 314(May 1, 1986): 1160–1163.

27. Howell, "Low Income Persons' Access to Health Care," pp. 507–516.

28. Brown, "Medicare and Medicaid," pp. 335–336.

29. K. Davis, G. Anderson, D. Rowland, and E. Steinberg, *Health Care Cost Containment* (Baltimore, Md.: The Johns Hopkins University Press, 1990).

30. Wilensky and Berk, "Health Care, the Poor and the Role of Medicaid," pp. 93–106.

31. J. Feder, J. Hadley, and R. Mullner, "Falling Through the Cracks: Poverty, Insurance Coverage, and Hospital Care for the Poor, 1980–1982," *Milbank Memorial Fund Quarterly/Health and Society* 62(1984): 544–566.

32. Kleinman, Gold, and Makuc, "Use of Ambulatory Medical Care by the Poor," pp. 1011–1029.

33. Howell, "Low Income Persons' Access to Health Care," pp. 507–516.

34. S. Jencks and B. Benedict, "Accessibility and Effectiveness of Care Under Medicaid," *Health Care Financing Review* (1990): 47–56.

35. J. Mitchell, "Physician Participation under Medicaid Revisited," *Medical Care* 29(July 1991):645–653.

36. American Medical Association, "Physician Participation in Medicaid," *Physician Marketplace Update* 2(July 1991).

37. Physician Payment Review Commission, *Annual Report to Congress*, 1991.

38. M. McManus, S. Flint, and R. Kelly, "The Adequacies of Physician Reimbursement for Pediatric Care Under Medicaid," *Pediatrics* 87(June 1991):909–920.

39. Physician Payment Review Commission, *Annual Report to Congress*, 1991.

40. Davis, "Achievements and Problems of Medicaid," pp. 309–316; Rogers, Blendon, and Moloney, "Who Needs Medicaid," pp. 13–18; Davis and Schoen, *Health and the War on Poverty.*

41. J. Hadley, *More Medical Care, Better Health* (Washington, D.C.: Urban Institute, 1982).

42. N. Lurie, N. Ward, M. Shapiro, and R. Brook, "Termination from Medi-Cal: Does It Affect Health?" *New England Journal of Medicine* 311(August 16, 1984):480–484; N. Lurie, N. Ward, M. Shapiro, R. Vaghaiwalla, and R. Brook, "Termination of Medi-Cal Benefits: A Follow-Up Study One Year Later," *New England Journal of Medicine* 314(May 8,1986):1266–1268.

43. P. Braveman, G. Oliva, M. G. Miller, R. Reiter, and S. Egerter, "Adverse Outcomes and Lack of Health Insurance Among Newborns in an Eight-County Area of California, 1982–1986," *New England Journal of Medicine* 321(August 24; 1989):508–512.

44. Hadley, Steinberg, and Feder, "Comparison of Uninsured and Privately Insured Hospital Patients," pp. 374–379.

45. D. Rowland, B. Lyons, and J. Edwards, "Medicaid: Health Care for the Poor in the Reagan Era," *Annual Review of Public Health* 9(1988):427–450; M. McManus and S. Davidson, "Medicaid as Public Health Insurance for Children," in M. J. Schlesinger and L. Eisenberg, eds., *Children in a Changing Health System: Assessments and Proposals for Reform* (Baltimore, Md.: Johns Hopkins University Press, 1990), pp. 131–157; Davis, "Achievements and Problems of Medicaid," pp. 309–316.

46. R. Blendon, L. Aiken, H. Freeman, B. Kirkman-Liff, and J. Murphy, "Uncompensated Care by Hospitals or Public Insurance for the Poor: Does it Make a Difference?" *New England Journal of Medicine* 314(May 1, 1986): 1160–1163.

47. Davis, "Achievements and Problems of Medicaid," pp. 309–316; Brown, "Medicare and Medicaid: the Process, Value and Limits of Health Care Reforms," pp. 335–336.

48. W. Cohen, "Reflections on the Enactment of Medicare and Medicaid," *Health Care Financing Review* (Annual Supplement, 1985):3–11.

49. Rowland, Lyons, and Edwards, "Medicaid," pp. 427–450.

50. H. Freeman, R. Blendon, L. Aiken, S. Sudman, C. Mullinix, and C. Corey, "Americans Report on Their Access to Care," *Health Affairs* 6(Spring 1987):6–18.

51. R. Blendon, "What Should Be Done About the Uninsured Poor?" *Journal of the American Medical Association* 260(December 2, 1987):3176–3177.

52. U.S. House of Representatives, Committee on Ways and Means, *The Green Book* (Washington, D.C.: Government Printing Office, 1991).

53. I. A. Merriam, Testimony at Hearing on Blue Cross and Other Private Health Insurance for the Elderly, U. S. Senate, Special Committee on Aging, Subcommittee on Health of the Elderly (Washington, D.C.: Government Printing Office, 1964), pp. 3–13.

54. K. Davis and D. Rowland, *Medicare Policy: New Directions for Health and Long Term Care* (Baltimore, Md.: The Johns Hopkins University Press, 1986).

55. Davis and Schoen, *Health and the War on Poverty,* pp. 18–49.

56. Davis and Schoen, *Health and the War on Poverty,* pp. 18–49; Brown, "Medicare and Medicaid," pp. 335–356.

57. K. Davis, "Equal Treatment and Unequal Benefits: The Medicare Program," *Milbank Memorial Fund Quarterly/Health and Society* (Fall 1975): 449–488; Davis and Rowland, *Medicare Policy: New Directions for Health and Long Term Care.*

58. L. A. Aday, R. Anderson, and G. Fleming, *Health Care in the U.S.: Equitable for Whom?* (Beverly Hills, Ca.: Sage Publications, 1980); Wilson and White, "Changes in Morbidity, Disability, and Utilization Differentials Between the Poor and the Nonpoor," pp. 636–646.

59. Aday, Anderson, and Fleming, *Health Care in the U.S.*.

60. Davis and Schoen, *Health and the War on Poverty,* pp. 18–49; Davis and Rowland, "Uninsured and Underserved," pp. 149–176.

61. K. Davis, "A Decade of Policy Developments in Providing Health Care to Low-Income Families," in R. Haveman, ed., *A Decade of Federal Anti-Poverty Policy: Achievements, Failures and Lessons* (New York, NY: Academic Press, 1977); Kleinman, Gold, and Makuc, "Use of Ambulatory Medical Care by the Poor: Another Look at Equity," pp. 1011–1029; Davis and Reynolds, "The Impact of Medicare and Medicaid on Access to Medical Care," pp. 391–425.

62. S. Long and R. F. Settle, "Medicare and the Disadvantaged Elderly: Objectives and Outcomes," *Milbank Memorial Fund Quarterly/Health and Society* 62(1984):609–656; Newacheck, "Access to Ambulatory Care for Poor Persons," pp. 401–419.

63. Davis and Reynolds, "The Impact of Medicare and Medicaid on Access to Medical Care," pp. 391–425.

64. Newacheck, "Access to Ambulatory Care for Poor Persons," pp. 401–419.

65. Blendon, Aiken, Freeman, Kirkman-Liff, and Murphy, "Uncompensated Care by Hospitals or Public Insurance for the Poor," pp. 1160–1163.

66. U.S. Congressional Budget Office, Updated Estimates of Medicare's Catastrophic Drug Insurance Program (October 1989).

67. S. Long, R. Settle, and C. Link, "Who Bears the Burden of Medicare Cost Sharing?" *Inquiry* 19(Fall 1982):222–234; C. Link, S. Long, and R. Settle, "Costsharing, Supplementary Insurance, and Health Services Utilization Among the Medicare Elderly," *Health Care Financing Review* 2(Fall 1980):25–31; Davis and Schoen, *Health and the War on Poverty,* pp. 18–49.

68. J. Feder, M. Moon, and W. Scanlon, "Medicare Reform: Nibbling at Catastrophic Costs," *Health Affairs* (Fall 1987):5–19.

69. D. Rowland, "Fewer Resources, Greater Burdens: Medical Care Coverage for Low-Income Elderly People," prepared for the U.S. Bipartisan Commission on Comprehensive Health Care (Washington, D.C.: Government Printing Office, 1990).

70. Rowland, "Fewer Resources, Greater Burdens," pp. 125–145.

71. Rowland, "Fewer Resources, Greater Burdens," pp. 125–145.

72. The Commonwealth Fund, *Medicare's Poor: Filling the Gaps in Medical Coverage for Low-Income Elderly Americans,* Report of the Commonwealth Fund Commission on Elderly People Living Alone (November, 1987).

73. J. Feder, "Health Care of the Disadvantaged: The Elderly," *Health Care of the Disadvantaged* (1990):7–16.

Summary

David E. Rogers

This two-day conference devoted to the subject of medical care and the health of the poor produced searching, indeed sometimes searing, discussions. Rarely at these conferences has there been such a consensus about the severity and the human costs of a problem. Unanimous was the feeling that the U.S. health care system seriously fails too many of its citizens at the bottom of the economic ladder. Furthermore, and adding to the intensity of the dialogue, was the agreement that the system was also badly out of synchrony with the hopes and the needs of the rest of the population as well. Despite Julius Richmond's gentle reminders that we had done a great deal to strengthen our health care system since World War II (he pointed to the enormous increases in resources allocated, vast additions to numbers of health professionals, the passage of Medicare and Medicaid, and the creation of the National Health Service Corps, neighborhood health centers, and Head Start), little good was said about what had evolved.

To give the reader some flavor of the criticisms, here were some of the things that were said about it. "A system out of control..." "Unacceptably expensive and becoming more so..." "Too high technology oriented..." "Dreadfully designed to deal with long term chronic relapsing illnesses..." "Leaves too many people out..." "Seriously lacking in primary or generalist care..." "Too hospital based..." "Too lacking in preventative health care services..." "Too medically oriented..." "Dominated by rapacious insurance companies that have lost their sense of community responsibility or willingness to risk share..."

It was also brought out that other groups in society that were not represented at the conference had similar views. The increasing frustrations of corporate executives who complain of uncontrollable costs and their impact on the competitiveness of U.S. businesses in world markets; the surprising recent election of Harris Wofford to the U.S. Senate from Pennsylvania, whose views on health care reform helped carry him to victory; and the swift rise to the top of many recent polls of worries about the costs and character of medical care pointed to broad dissatisfactions with what has come to pass.

On the specific problem of medical care and the health of the poor, no one disputed the basic and long-recognized correlation: When taken in the aggregate, the poorer a person is, the worse her or his health status is. But despite that tight association, much remained uncertain about precise causality factors. Victor Fuchs's thoughtful discussion prompted a careful look at this association, pointing out that poverty might be a proxy for other attitudes or behaviors leading to illness and poor health. David Mechanic indicated that although health status correlates most precisely with years of education, the "why" remains unclear. These uncertainties were reinforced by Douglas Black's report on what had happened to health in Britain under 30 years of universal entitlement and more equitable availability of health care services. Despite notable improvements in overall morbidity and mortality, the differences in the health status of the five British occupational classes remained great. Indeed, differences were actually larger than before the introduction of the National Health Service! Thus, Black preferred to simply link poor health with what he labeled "social deprivation."

Conferees were also unanimous in their view that the social and economic costs of the disturbing health status of many of the poor were a serious impediment to the future. Considerable evidence was advanced to suggest that directing resources at relieving social deprivation resulted in the most noticeable improvements in health. Perhaps most powerful was the evidence presented by Arden Miller that income supplementation, family planning, and the Head Start programs had materially improved the health outcomes for children touched by these efforts.

The other side of the coin—whether medical care could itself materially improve the health of the poor—was examined by Nicole Lurie and Mary Charlson. Both presented convincing data that in the case of certain disease conditions where effective medical interventions were available (they chose diabetes, hypertension, and arthritis), medical care could improve health even in the absence of dramatic changes in socioeconomic status. Margaret Hamburg's moving luncheon talk showed that tuberculosis—a disease now looming large in New York City—was yet another illness in which the strength of our medical technologies was such that simple administration of antituberculosis drugs could cure this disease without changes in income, housing, or any of the other social conditions desirable for a better quality of life.

But in the main, it was agreed that improving the health of poor people seemed best addressed by measures more social and economic than medical. The importance of adequate income, education, housing, and stable human and community support systems was repeatedly stressed. None of these seemed easily available for low-income citizens in the United States today. Indeed, many felt that the social programs that had yielded positive results during the 1960s and 1970s had been largely dismantled during the 1980s. As vividly presented by Paul Starr, a democracy can indeed tolerate a fair amount of inequity in its arrangements for health care. But none of the participants felt that the current situation, which leaves so many of the poor outside of a health care system, is acceptable. The gap is too wide.

A considerable amount of the discussion focused on the obvious question "If things are so bad, why have we not moved more swiftly to correct these inequities?" Among the reasons advanced were the deep-seated and increasing American distrust of central government, public worries that any change in the system designed to better include low-income groups would add even more in costs, worries that solutions answering the needs of one group would reduce the availability of services for others, and what Victor Fuchs delicately called the "weakness of our noblesse oblige." Others translated this to mean the increasing selfishness of Americans during tough economic times.

But there was yet one other area of general agreement that added to a collective feeling of urgency—namely, that a level of national discontent, anger, insecurity, fear, and dissatisfaction about health care was now sufficiently widespread as to permit significant change to be made if energies were properly directed. The majority of the conferees felt the time was ripe to once again move toward some form of universal entitlement—a national system of financing health care for all. This would require a skillful blending of public and private mechanisms to be successful. This mix had one important proviso: that the public part be large. Victor Fuchs's figure showing two models of a two-tiered system provoked much continuing discussion. Most agreed that any system should look more like that portrayed in column B, with a large second tier. All agreed that two tiers would be acceptable only with Paul Starr's ground rule—that the second tier be constructed with sufficient generosity that all of us would be willing to be included within it. A program designed only for the poor was believed destined to fail, and this view was strengthened by Diane Rowland's discussion. As clearly illustrated by her contribution, Medicare was socially acceptable by all and popular with the recipients in large measure because it was universal in coverage and was working well. Medicaid was unpopular, was generally regarded negatively and associated with welfare, was viewed as taking dollars out of every citizen's pocket for the benefit of one special group, and was working poorly. To get the poor into a sustainable system of health care required the use of an inclusionary strategy and of a program that was universally applied, simple, and easily understood. It was agreed that any system of care must link the middle class and the rest of us to the poor if it is to be broadly accepted. As Diane Rowland noted, "To help the poor, we must do it without talking about them."

The last compelling reason for believing that this was the time to push for a universal financing mechanism was the view that this was the only way to get a handle on the skyrocketing costs of health care. It was Victor Fuchs's belief, shared by all, that only if we could get "upstream resource control"—caps on the numbers of physicians, the numbers of hospitals, the supply of resources utilized—could we gain control of health care costs. Furthermore, only by preventing the relentless increase in medical care costs could funds be freed up to address other pressing social needs, such as education or housing, and those social programs that have a profound influence on health.

While all wished to move toward some form of universal financing for health care, many modifications and variations on this theme were suggested. The establishment of a protected trust fund for health services for children was advanced. (Some felt that coverage of children should be mandatory in any program.) Fitzhugh Mullan felt that more careful attention to the personnel needs—the nature of the physician and the other kinds of health professionals—that make for a more responsive and less costly system should be tied to financing. Some suggested that the states be permitted to initiate universal coverage rather than having the responsibilities placed immediately with the federal sector. Most felt that resources for tertiary care should be limited and redistributed in a system that emphasized generalist out-of-hospital care. Toward the end of the conference, many felt that marching under the banner "MEDICARE FOR ALL" with buyouts to allow supplemental coverage would be the most appropriate and readily understood message to send at this time. Clear was the need to design a program so that the vast majority of people, who felt happy with their current health care arrangements, would not feel threatened.

But there were doubters. Eli Ginzberg felt that the economic realities of the present, the magnitude of the dollars required, and the attitudinal shifts that would be asked of the majority of Americans to put any form of universal coverage in place were beyond what could be expected. Indeed, at his most provocative he stated that the situation would have to go "from crisis to chaos—that the system would have to be totally derailed" before Americans would be willing to make the sacrifices necessary to put a more equitable and responsive health care system in place. His views are forcibly outlined in the overview.

But at closure all were agreed that our current health care system is in serious trouble. Its costs, both economically and socially, are viewed as unacceptable by more Americans than perhaps ever before. Its failure to reach too many of the "socially deprived" in our society is being felt ever more widely and is a source of increasing national discomfort and embarrassment. Most participants believed that the current unhappiness with the system may have created a "window of opportunity" for change. To get at the problem of those left out, all agreed we must focus on the wishes, hopes, and aspirations of the majority—the middle class—for its health care. Clearly we must not be too doctrinaire in the design of universal financing mechanisms. We are too diverse a people. We must use inclusionary, not exclusionary, strategies. All too clear are the enormous human and fiscal obstacles to constructive change. Nevertheless, we must recognize that most major reforms in social systems have had to overcome continuing political cynicism. To do so requires evangelistic optimists. We need articulate, discontented, caring people to push for a better world. A number of them were present at this conference.

About the Contributors

John P. Allegrante, Ph.D., is Associate Professor of Health Education and of Clinical Public Health in Sociomedical Sciences, Columbia University, and Associate Director of the Education, Epidemiology and Health Services Research Component, Cornell Arthritis and Musculoskeletal Disease Center, The Hospital for Special Surgery.

Douglas Black is former president, Royal College of Physicians, London.

Mary E. Charlson, M.D., is Associate Professor of Medicine, The New York Hospital-Cornell Medical Center.

Victor R. Fuchs, Ph.D., is Henry J. Kaiser, Jr. Professor, Stanford University and Research Associate, National Bureau of Economic Research.

Eli Ginzberg, Ph.D., is Professor Emeritus, School of Business, Columbia University, and Director, The Eisenhower Center for the Conservation of Human Resources, Columbia University.

Margaret A. Hamburg, M.D., is Commissioner of Health, the City of New York.

Nicole Lurie, M.D., MSPH, is Associate Professor Medicine and Director of Clinical Epidemiology, University of Minnesota.

C. Arden Miller, M.D., is Professor of Maternal and Child Health, School of Public Health, The University of North Carolina at Chapel Hill.

Laura Robbins, ACSW, is Director, Department of Community Education, The Hospital for Special Surgery, and Associate Director of Educational Research and Development, Cornell Arthritis and Musculoskeletal Disease Center.

David E. Rogers, M.D., is The Walsh McDermott University Professor of Medicine, Cornell University Medical College.

Diane Rowland, Sc.D., is Assistant Professor, School of Hygiene and Public Health, The Johns Hopkins University and Executive Director, Kaiser Commission on the Future of Medicaid.

Paul Starr, Ph.D., is Professor of Sociology, Princeton University.

Cornell University Medical College Eighth Conference on Health Policy

Medical Care and the Health of the Poor
February 21–28, 1992, New York, New York

Conference Co-Chairmen

David E. Rogers, M.D.
The Walsh McDermott University Professor of Medicine
Cornell University Medical College

Eli Ginzberg, Ph.D.
Director
The Eisenhower Center for the Conservation of Human Resources
Columbia University

Conference Coordinator

Ms. Diane Rothschild Arditti
Cornell University Medical College

Speakers

Sir Douglas Black
Former President, Royal College of Physicians of London

Mary E. Charlson, M.D.
Associate Professor of Medicine
The New York Hospital-Cornell Medical Center

Victor R. Fuchs, Ph.D.
Professor of Economics
Stanford University

Margaret Hamburg, M.D.
Commissioner of Health
New York City

Nicole Lurie, M.D., MSPH
Associate Professor of Medicine and Director of Clinical Epidemiology
University of Minnesota

C. Arden Miller, M.D.
Professor of Maternal and Child Health
School of Public Health
University of North Carolina

Cesar Perales
Deputy Mayor, New York City
Office of Health and Human Services

Diane Rowland, Sc.D.
Assistant Professor
School of Hygiene and Public Health
Johns Hopkins University

Paul Starr, Ph.D.
Professor of Sociology
Princeton University

Participants

Jeremiah A. Barondess, M.D.
President
New York Academy of Medicine

Richard Behrman, M.D.
Managing Director
Center for the Future of Children
David and Lucille Packard Foundation

Barbara Blum
President
Foundation for Child Development

Morton Bogdonoff, M.D.
Professor of Medicine
The New York Hospital-Cornell Medical Center

Robert Braham, M.D.
Associate Chairman for Clinical Services
Department of Medicine
The New York Hospital-Cornell Medical Center

Philip Brickner, M.D.
Director, Department of Community Medicine
St. Vincent's Hospital

Karon Davis, Ph.D.
Professor and Chair
Department of Health Policy and Management
Johns Hopkins University

Rashi Fein, Ph.D.
Professor of the Economics of Medicine
Harvard Medical School

Jack Hadley, Ph.D.
Co-Director
Center for Health Policy Studies
Georgetown University

Karen Hein, M.D.
Director, Adolescent AIDS Program
Department of Pediatrics
Montefiore Medical Center

Margaret Hilgartner, M.D.
Professor of Pediatrics
The New York Hospital-Cornell Medical Center

Judith E. Jones, M.S.
Director, The National Center for Children in Poverty
Associate Clinical Professor of Public Health
Columbia University School of Public Health

Sol Levine, Ph.D.
Director, Society and Health Program
New England Medical Center

James A. Marone, Ph.D.
Associate Professor, Political Science
Brown University

David Mechanic, Ph.D.
University Professor
Institute for Health
Rutgers University

Thomas W. Moloney
Senior Vice President
The Commonwealth Fund

Fitzhugh Mullan, M.D.
Director, Bureau of Health Professions
Assistant Surgeon General
Public Health Service

Alicia H. Munnell
Senior Vice President and Director of Research
Federal Reserve Bank of Boston

Karen Nelson
Staff Director for Subcommittee on Health and Environment
U.S. House of Representatives

Irwin Redlener, M.D.
Chief of Community Pediatrics
Montefiore Medical Center

Julius B. Richmond, M.D.
Professor of Health Policy
Harvard Medical School

Mark Smith, M.D.
Vice President
The Henry J. Kaiser Foundation

Alvin R. Tarlov, M.D.
Director, Division of Health Improvements and Senior Scientist
New England Medical Center

Index